HEART
HEALTHY
FOR LIFE

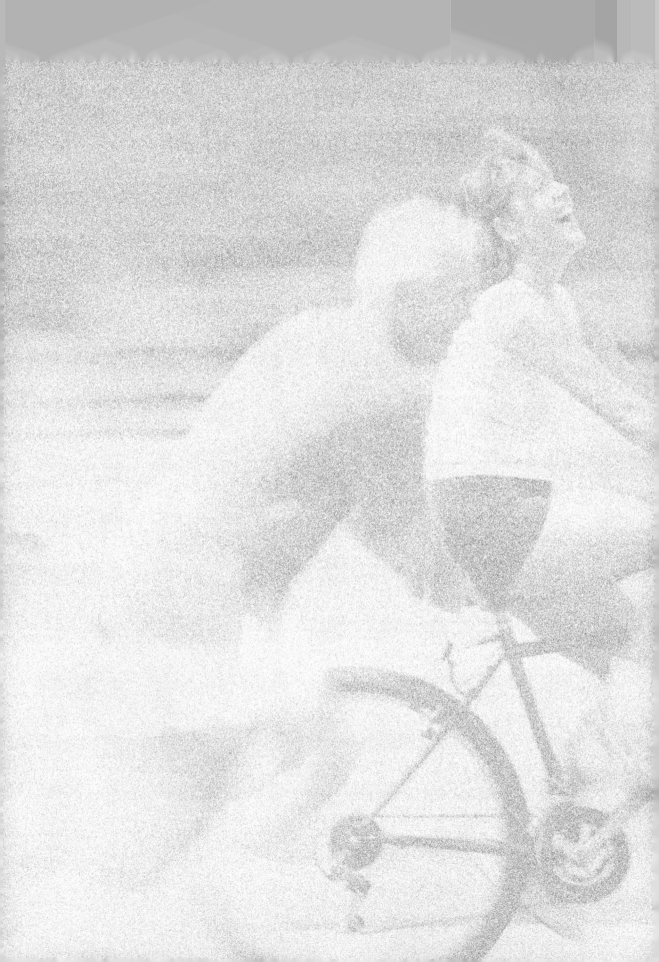

HEART HEALTHY FOR LIFE

Peter Jaret

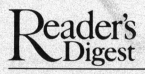

Reader's Digest

The Reader's Digest Association, Inc., Pleasantville, New York/Montreal

READER'S DIGEST PROJECT STAFF

Senior Editor
Marianne Wait

Senior Designer
Judith Carmel

Production Technology Manager
Douglas A. Croll

CONTRIBUTORS

Writer
Peter Jaret

Design
Nina Scerbo Design Inc.

Copy Editor
Carol Mauro-Noon

Indexer
Nanette Bendyna

MEDICAL CONSULTANT

Rita F. Redberg, M.D., M.Sc.
Associate Professor of Medicine,
University of California San
Francisco School of Medicine,
Division of Cardiology

READER'S DIGEST HEALTH PUBLISHING

Editorial Director
Neil Wertheimer

Marketing Director
James H. Malloy

Vice President and General Manager
Shirrel Rhoades

THE READER'S DIGEST ASSOCIATION, INC.

Editor-in-Chief
Eric W. Schrier

President, North American Books and Home Entertainment
Thomas D. Gardner

Library of Congress Cataloging in Publication Data

Jaret, Peter.
   Heart healthy for life/Peter Jaret.
     p. cm.
   Includes index.
   ISBN 0-7621-0397-3 (hardcover)
   ISBN 0-7621-0452-X (paperback)
    1. Coronary heart disease—Popular works. I. Title.

RC685.C6 J37 2002
616.1'23—dc21   2002022728

Address any comments about *Heart Healthy for Life* to:
Reader's Digest
Editorial Director, Reader's Digest Health Publishing
Reader's Digest Road
Pleasantville, NY 10570

To order additional copies of *Heart Healthy for Life*,
call 1-800-846-2100.

Visit our website at rd.com

Printed in the United States of America.

1 3 5 7 9 10 8 6 4 2 (hardcover)
1 3 5 7 9 10 8 6 4 2 (paperback)

Note to Readers
The information in this book should not be substituted for, or used to alter, medical therapy without your doctor's advice. For a specific health problem, consult your physician for guidance.

US 3913H/IC

About This Book

Unlike some diseases, which doctors have no clue how to prevent, heart disease is almost entirely avoidable. Even if you've already been diagnosed with heart disease, you can significantly lower your risk of having a heart attack.

You probably knew that. But exactly how do you go about it? Do you have to eliminate fat from your diet? (Definitely not.) How much exercise is enough? (Probably less than you think.) Why bother changing your lifestyle at all when a pill can bring your cholesterol down and lower your blood pressure?

You'll discover the answers to these questions and dozens more in **HEART HEALTHY FOR LIFE.** Better still, you'll find out how to take small, easy steps that have been proven to lower the risk of dying from heart disease. Remember, the condition is downright rare in certain parts of the world where people eat differently, exercise more, and live with less stress. In other words, the health of your heart is in your hands.

This book is for you if you've been diagnosed with coronary artery disease. It's also for you if you have risk factors such as high blood pressure, elevated cholesterol, or a family history of heart attacks. In these pages you'll find an abundance of practical advice, all based on the very latest research. Learn why nuts are good for you—even if you're trying to lose weight. Find out how deep-breathing exercises can help lower your blood pressure. Discover a simple gadget you can use to motivate you to exercise more. Because heart disease sometimes requires medical intervention, you'll also read important information about the newest drugs and surgical techniques.

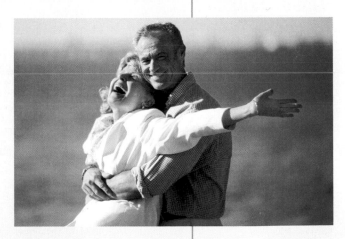

We know that change is hard. That's why you'll hear from behavioral experts on how to break out of old routines successfully. Look for the "Real People, Real Wisdom" features for inspiration from people just like you who've faced challenges and come out on top. Finally, turn to page 222 for a core collection of more than three dozen heart smart recipes to start you on your way to a longer, healthier, more enjoyable life.

Foreword

Rita F. Redberg, M.D., M.Sc.

The past decade has witnessed tremendous strides in understanding and treating heart disease. State-of-the-art tools help us better diagnose everything from abnormal heart rhythms to blockages in the arteries that supply blood to the heart. When we detect a problem, we can often treat it with powerful new drugs or remarkably precise surgical procedures. We can open up clogged arteries or bypass them completely. Best of all, we now know how most cases of heart disease can be prevented.

Despite all this good news, however, heart disease remains the number one killer in the United States. And men aren't the only victims. Although most women worry more about breast cancer, far more women (one in three) will die of cardiovascular disease (diseases of the heart and blood vessels, including conditions that cause strokes).

Why does heart disease still take such a deadly toll? The reasons are many. First, it's easy to be unaware of the disease, partly because symptoms aren't often obvious in the early stages. In fact, many people don't know they have a problem until they suffer a heart attack. Also, lifestyle has a lot to do with heart disease risk—and unfortunately, many of us still put our hearts in danger because of the way we live. Too much fatty food, too little exercise, too much stress, bad habits like cigarette smoking—all of them add up to potential trouble.

The vast majority of heart attacks don't have to happen. As I tell many of my patients, the most effective ways to avoid heart problems—or to lower the danger of having a heart attack if you have coronary artery disease—are things you can do on your own.

HEART HEALTHY FOR LIFE gives you a wealth of practical strategies to protect yourself. Put even some of them into practice, and you're likely to add years to your life. Research shows that by cutting down on saturated fat in your diet, for instance, you can lower your risk of heart attack by at least 50 percent. This book contains dozens of tips for making your diet—and the rest of your lifestyle—more heart friendly.

If your heart is healthy, making these changes will help keep it that way. If you already have heart disease, they can go a long way

> " The most effective ways to avoid heart problems—or to lower the danger of having a heart attack if you have coronary artery disease—are things you can do on your own. "

toward reversing it. Of course, cardiologists like me often have to treat patients with drugs or surgical procedures. We have medications that are remarkably effective at lowering cholesterol or preventing the blood clots that can lead to heart attacks, as well as pills that lower blood pressure or ease the burden on weakened hearts. But even our best treatments aren't as powerful as the strategies in this book.

Believe me, I know that embarking on a heart healthy life takes real commitment. And that commitment usually comes from believing in the power of what you're doing. In my practice, I find that most patients will accept the idea that a medication will help them. Some people even think they've done something good for their hearts just by getting a test. But many of them aren't quite convinced that eating less saturated fat or getting more exercise will make a big difference to their health. By explaining exactly how factors such as diet, exercise, and stress management affect your heart, **HEART HEALTHY FOR LIFE** will help convince you that changing a few habits is well worth the effort.

I've seen the power of prevention firsthand. One of my patients didn't know she had coronary artery disease until she suffered a heart attack and had to undergo an angioplasty, a technique used to open up blocked arteries. Another patient had a heart attack in his sixties. Both of them were very scared. And both of them made up their minds right away that they weren't going to end up in the hospital again. She really focused on her diet, filling the refrigerator with fruits and vegetables and trying new heart healthy recipes. He concentrated on exercise, setting up a gym in his study, where he still exercises every morning for half an hour. Both of them have now gone for at least five years without any more heart problems.

They also tell me they feel better. They have more energy. They have a more positive outlook. I think they even have a greater sense of self-esteem. Those changes aren't easy for doctors to measure with blood tests or electrodes. But they are some of the real rewards you'll gain by following the advice in this book.

Contents

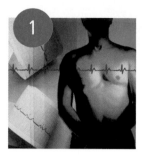
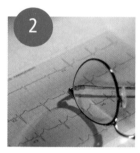
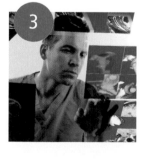
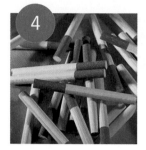
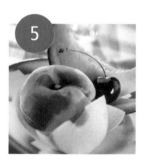
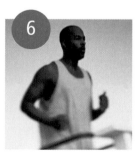

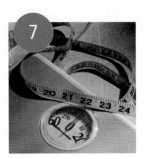
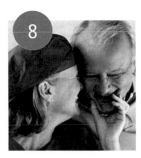
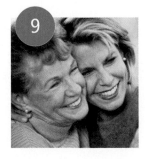
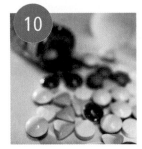
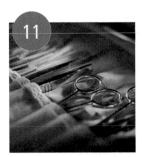
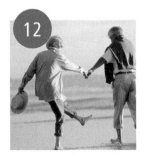

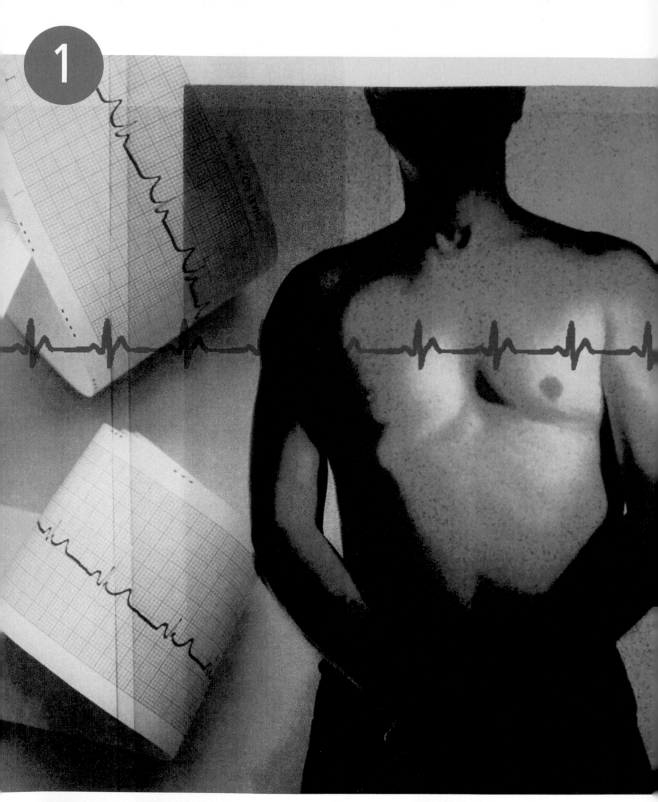

The Heart of the Matter

First, it's time for a little pat on the back. Since 1950, when health experts sounded the alarm about a rising epidemic of heart attacks among Americans, the rate of heart disease in the United States has fallen by almost 60 percent. The U.S. Centers for Disease Control and Prevention recently called this decline "one of the most important public health achievements of the 20th century."

So, good for us. And now it's time to do even better.

Despite the progress we've made, cardiovascular disease remains the single most serious health threat Americans face. More Americans die of it today than of any other illness. Cardiovascular disease, which includes diseases of the heart or blood vessels, kills more people than the next seven causes of death combined. The most common heart-related illness, called coronary artery disease, causes more deaths than all types of cancer combined. And recently, experts have noted a worrisome uptick in the rate of heart attacks.

An estimated 60 million Americans suffer from some form of cardiovascular disease. One million Americans are expected to die from it this year alone. That's 26,000 deaths every day caused by diseases related to the heart and circulatory system.

But there's good news, too. Heart disease isn't inevitable. In fact, it's one of the most preventable of all serious illnesses.

> Despite the progress we've made, cardiovascular disease remains the single most serious health threat Americans face.

You're in Control

By making a few doable changes in your daily routine, you can dramatically reduce your risk of heart attack. If you've already had one, you can avoid having another. And you don't have to turn your life upside down to do it. Take a brisk walk after dinner in place of watching one sitcom on most nights of the week, and you've already started to arm yourself against trouble. Trim a bit of saturated fat from your menu, and you'll compound that protection. If you smoke, muster the courage to quit, and you'll slash your risk of heart disease in half.

There's plenty your doctor can do, too. Thanks to advances in treatment, the prospects of living a long and active life even if you've been diagnosed with advanced heart disease are better than ever before. New medications can lower elevated cholesterol and high blood pressure, helping to keep heart attacks and strokes at bay. Sophisticated surgical techniques are repairing blocked arteries and fixing damage to the heart itself.

We know more today than even 10 years ago about what keeps a heart healthy, what makes it sick, and how to make it better. *Heart Healthy for Life* will put this knowledge in your hands.

Your heart, in health and sickness

The human heart beats an average of 70 times a minute, 4,200 times an hour, 100,800 times a day. With each beat, this muscular pump pushes blood through a complex network of blood vessels that if laid end to end would stretch 60,000 miles. Clearly, the heart is a pretty tough organ. Yet plenty of things can go wrong.

PROGRESS ON MANY FRONTS

What explains the dramatic decline in heart disease rates over the past 50 years? Surprisingly, researchers aren't sure. So much progress has been made in so many areas of heart disease prevention that it's likely that many changes have contributed.

Still, it's important for researchers to know what works and what doesn't in order to focus public health efforts. Not long ago, scientists from the Harvard School of Public Health analyzed a decade's worth of heart disease data from around the country. They estimated that 25 percent of the decline in

Americans are eating less saturated fat—one reason heart disease in the United States is on the wane.

coronary artery disease resulted from primary prevention efforts geared to keep healthy people from developing heart problems, such as the push to lower the amount of saturated fat in our diets. An additional 29 percent was explained by secondary prevention efforts, those aimed at reducing risk factors like high blood pressure and elevated cholesterol in people already diagnosed with heart trouble. And 43 percent was attributed to advances in treatments, such as bypass surgery and techniques to repair blocked arteries.

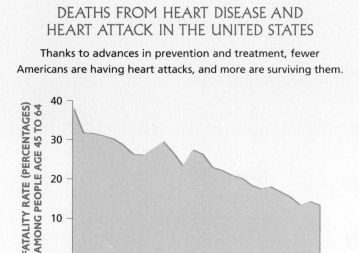

DEATHS FROM HEART DISEASE AND
HEART ATTACK IN THE UNITED STATES

Thanks to advances in prevention and treatment, fewer
Americans are having heart attacks, and more are surviving them.

FATALITY RATE (PERCENTAGES)
AMONG PEOPLE AGE 45 TO 64

Source: The National Center for Health Statistics and the National
Heart, Lung, and Blood Institute

Heart disease takes many forms, from congenital defects in heart valves to infections that damage heart muscles. Far and away the greatest threat comes from a process called atherosclerosis, or hardening of the arteries. And the chief culprit is serum cholesterol, a waxy substance that circulates through the blood.

Over time, cholesterol can build up to form deposits inside blood vessel walls. Like sediment in water pipes, these deposits may restrict blood flow. Eventually blockages can form. When the coronary arteries, which supply blood to the heart, become obstructed, the result is coronary artery disease, the leading cause of heart attacks. When vessels in the neck that supply blood to the brain narrow, carotid artery disease results. If the blockage becomes bad enough, portions of the brain can be robbed of the blood and oxygen they need, causing a stroke.

Too much of a good thing

Here's more proof that heart disease isn't inevitable: A century ago heart attacks were uncommon in many parts of the world. Even today, rates of heart disease vary widely from country to country.

Why has cardiovascular disease become the number one killer in the United States? In a sense, we are the victims of our own good fortune. Laborsaving devices have taken over most hard physical

FAST FACT

Americans today

consume an average of

14 pounds less red meat

and 3.5 pounds more

fish per year than they

did in 1970.

work. Food manufacturers have filled our tables with an array of tempting choices. At the same time, the demands of modern life seem to cause unprecedented pressure. This combination of abundant food (much of it laden with fat), sedentary lifestyles, and unrelenting stress can spell big trouble for our hearts.

Because cardiovascular disease is associated with rich diets and sedentary living, it is sometimes called a disease of affluence. But that term may be misleading. It's true that the risk is generally higher in many industrialized societies than in some less developed societies, partly because traditional diets are often healthier than diets centered on processed foods. Within the United States, however, heart disease strikes people at every socioeconomic level.

Key Finding

Adopting some new habits really can save your life, according to recent results from the Nurses' Health Study. Among more than 84,000 nurses, those who didn't smoke, who followed a heart healthy diet, and who exercised regularly were 80 percent less likely than those with less healthy lifestyles to have a heart attack during a 14-year period of study.

The Heart Healthy approach

Heart Healthy for Life offers an action plan that will shore up your heart and circulatory system against future problems and even reverse some of the signs and symptoms of heart disease. Is it worth the work? You bet. Consider this: Making just five lifestyle changes, research shows, could prevent as many as four out of five cases of coronary artery disease. The same five changes will keep you healthier if you've already been diagnosed with heart problems.

1. Kick the habit. If you smoke, we're going to join the chorus of voices encouraging you to quit—and we're going to show you how. Smoking is deadly for many reasons. Chemicals in cigarette smoke restrict the flow of blood and make blood cells called platelets stickier than normal, increasing the risk of a dangerous blood clot. Carbon monoxide from cigarette smoke reduces the amount of oxygen that reaches your heart. Kick the habit, and you'll start reaping the health benefits the moment you do.

2. Get moving. Believe it or not, being a couch potato can be every bit as dangerous to your heart as smoking. If your idea of exercise is reaching for the remote control, don't worry. Becoming even moderately active—nothing more strenuous than 30 minutes of brisk walking most days of the week—could slash your chances of having a heart attack almost in half. We'll explain how

TALE OF A CITY

"In 1948, we didn't pay much attention to what we were eating," recalls Walter Sullivan, 87, a retired lawyer who lives in Massachusetts. "My favorite breakfast was eggs and bacon. My wife, Katie, and I smoked. We never exercised."

That year the Sullivans volunteered to participate in a bold medical experiment being organized in their hometown of Framingham. Alarmed by the growing epidemic of heart disease in the United States, scientists from the U.S. Public Health Service recruited more than 5,000 healthy residents ages 30 to 60 from Framingham. Every two years the volunteers received a careful medical examination and a battery of tests. By analyzing the data, researchers hoped to find clues to the causes of heart disease.

The Framingham Heart Study has been running for more than half a century. More than 20,000 people have participated. The Sullivans (and now their children) still go in for regular exams. Thanks to them, the study has made dozens of lifesaving discoveries. Here are some of the landmark findings.

1957 High blood pressure and high cholesterol levels linked to heart disease risk

1961 Researchers coin the term "risk factor"

1962 Cigarette smoking shown to increase risk of heart disease

1967 Physical activity found to lower cardiovascular disease risk

1970 High blood pressure linked to increased risk of stroke

1974 Diabetes linked to cardiovascular disease danger

1977 Experts describe the effects of triglycerides, low-density lipoproteins (LDL cholesterol) and high-density lipoproteins (HDL cholesterol) on heart disease risk

1981 Filter cigarettes shown to offer no protection against heart disease

1988 High levels of HDL cholesterol shown to reduce cardiovascular disease risk

1997 Researchers describe the cumulative effects of smoking, high blood pressure, and high cholesterol on heart disease

1998 Gene linked to high blood pressure discovered

Today, the researchers are investigating genetic links to heart disease and exploring other risk factors that may provide early warning signs of trouble.

These days, Walter Sullivan is much more careful about his diet, thanks to the findings he and his family helped generate. "Eggs are a special treat now. I eat more fish and less beef than before. Most days of the week I spend half an hour riding an exercise bicycle and working with free weights. And of course we gave up smoking a long time ago." At 87 he still gardens in the spring, rakes leaves in the fall, and shovels snow in the winter—a testament to the benefits of a heart-healthy lifestyle.

Top 10 Causes of Death in the United States

1. Heart disease
2. Cancer
3. Stroke
4. Chronic obstructive pulmonary disease
5. Accidents
6. Pneumonia/ Influenza
7. Diabetes
8. Suicide
9. Nephritis, nephrotic syndrome, and nephrosis
10. Chronic liver disease and cirrhosis

Source: National Center for Health Statistics

buying a simple device called a step counter can spur your exercise efforts and keep you on track.

3. Eat smart. No, we don't mean sitting down to a meal of bean sprouts and lentils every night. Or giving up the foods you love. Some of the world's most delicious cuisines—including the Mediterranean diet and the Asian diet—are also among the healthiest. By stealing a few of their secrets, you can guard your heart while treating your taste buds.

4. Slim down. At any given moment, half of all Americans say they want to lose weight. With good reason. High blood pressure, diabetes, and elevated cholesterol are linked to being overweight. Being moderately overweight increases your risk of heart disease. Being obese, or seriously overweight, is even more dangerous. If you've tried and failed to check that extra baggage, don't be discouraged: Shedding even a few pounds can make a positive difference for your heart. We'll show you how to cut calories without going hungry. Plus we'll tell you how you can boost your metabolism to burn more calories all day long and keep the weight off—permanently.

5. Relax. People who score high on tests that measure anger have been shown to run a higher risk of heart disease. And it's common for heart attacks to occur during stressful periods. Even if stress doesn't cause heart disease, a hectic day at the office or anxiety over problems at home can make it a lot harder for you to stick to your resolution to take that walk during your lunch hour or shun the jelly doughnut staring you in the face. Learning a few techniques to defuse anger and stress can help.

And Now for a Change ...

Thanks to more than 50 years of research, physicians today know the prescription for a healthy heart. So why aren't more people following it?

The reason is simple: Change isn't always easy. Modifying the way you eat—even just switching from whole milk to one percent, for example—requires a commitment. Something as seemingly feasible as walking 30 minutes a day on most days of the week can be difficult if you have a demanding schedule or you simply aren't used to exercising. And the prospect of quitting smoking can be downright daunting.

Eating heart smart can be a delicious endeavor. Are you ready to embark?

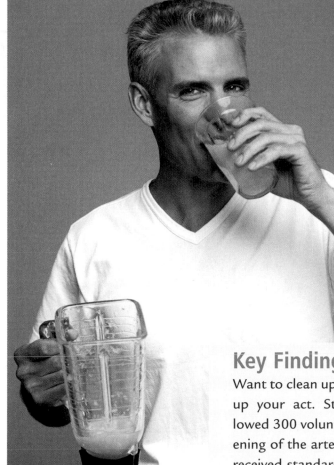

Key Finding

Want to clean up your arteries? You can—if you clean up your act. Stanford University researchers followed 300 volunteers, all with atherosclerosis (hardening of the arteries). Half were put in a group who received standard medical care. The other half were given a program of intensive counseling on improving their diet, exercising, and other heart-healthy lifestyles. Four years later, those who received the lifestyle counseling had a 47 percent lower rate of artery narrowing.

But you *can* do it. And psychologists who study how people make changes have gained a better understanding of what it takes. In *Heart Healthy for Life*, we'll share many of their insights to help smooth your way.

One crucial discovery is worth mentioning here. Whether you're trying to improve your diet, stop biting your fingernails, or become more active, experts have discovered that the process of change takes place in stages. According to James O. Prochaska, Ph.D., a professor of clinical and health psychology at the University of Rhode Island, there are five basic stages of change. If you're just beginning to think about tweaking your lifestyle to become heart healthy, for instance, you're at the "contemplation" stage. If you've been trying to make some changes and haven't

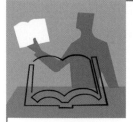

TERMS TO KNOW

ATHEROSCLEROSIS The medical term for hardening of the arteries, which is caused when deposits of fat, cholesterol, and other substances reduce the flow of blood through arteries

CARDIOVASCULAR DISEASE Any disease that affects the heart or the blood vessels

CAROTID ARTERY DISEASE Blockage of the neck arteries that supply the brain

CHOLESTEROL A waxy substance that in excess amounts can lead to atherosclerosis

CORONARY ARTERY DISEASE Blockage of the arteries that supply blood to the heart

HEART ATTACK (MYOCARDIAL INFARCTION) Damage to part of the heart muscle caused when a blockage in one of the coronary arteries robs heart tissue of blood and oxygen

PRIMARY PREVENTION Preventing the conditions that lead to heart disease, such as high blood pressure and elevated cholesterol

SECONDARY PREVENTION Preventing heart attacks or further cardiovascular damage in people already diagnosed with heart disease

STROKE Damage that occurs when an artery blockage robs the brain of blood and oxygen

quite succeeded yet, you're at a stage called "preparation."

Why does it matter? Because knowing your current stage of change can help you target strategies that will propel you to the next stage. Find out how ready you really are to get heart healthy by taking this short quiz. It examines just one aspect of your lifestyle—your diet. Circle the number beside the statement that most closely describes how you feel right now about making changes in the way you eat that could lower your risk of heart disease—cutting back on saturated fat, for instance, and eating more fruits, vegetables, and whole grains. Each of these statements corresponds to one of the five stages of change.

1. "To be honest, I'm just not willing to change at this point." (pre-contemplation)

2. "I think about trying to eat a healthier diet, but I haven't actually done anything about it yet." (contemplation)

3. "I do try now and then, but I just haven't been able to stick with it." (preparation)

4. "I recently began eating a healthier diet, and now my goal is to try to make my new habits stick." (action)

5. "I've been following a heart-healthy diet for six months or more already." (maintenance)

The statement you choose indicates how far along the path you are to making smart adjustments to your diet—one important step toward becoming heart healthy. Don't worry if you haven't come very far. Knowing where you stand now can help you focus on what you need to do to move forward. Next you'll find some basic strategies tailored to each of the five stages.

1. Precontemplation. If you're honestly not willing to change at this time, chances are you're not yet sure the benefits are worth the trouble. In *Heart Healthy for Life* we'll show you otherwise. Not only can adjusting your habits save your life, it will also make you feel better, look better, and have more energy to do the things you enjoy.

2. Contemplation. Just thinking about making positive changes represents a step forward. At this stage, it's important to begin making some practical plans to turn your good intention into action, such as buying a low-fat cookbook or resolving to help yourself to an extra serving of vegetables at dinner.

3. Preparation. If you've been trying to eat a healthier diet without much success, take a look at the obstacles that have gotten

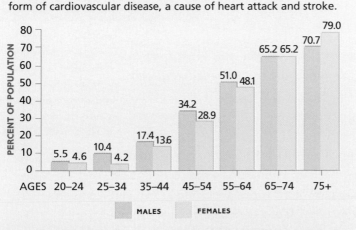

ESTIMATED PREVALENCE OF CARDIOVASCULAR DISEASE BY AGE AND SEX

By age 60 about half the U.S. population has developed some form of cardiovascular disease, a cause of heart attack and stroke.

AGES	MALES	FEMALES
20–24	5.5	4.6
25–34	10.4	4.2
35–44	17.4	13.6
45–54	34.2	28.9
55–64	51.0	48.1
65–74	65.2	65.2
75+	70.7	79.0

PERCENT OF POPULATION

Source: NHANES III (1988–1994), CDC/NCHS, and the American Heart Association

5 Myths About Heart Disease

1

Only men have heart attacks.
Wrong. Heart disease is the leading cause of death for women, too.

2

If heart disease runs in your family, there's not much you can do.
Even someone with a family history of the disease can do plenty to prevent a heart attack.

3

Heart disease is inevitable later in life.
Not so. In some parts of the world, heart disease is uncommon even among very old people.

4

The biggest danger from cigarette smoking is lung cancer.
In fact, the largest proportion of deaths related to smoking is due to heart disease.

5

If your cholesterol is normal, you don't need to worry about heart disease.
Cholesterol is only one of several risk factors, including high blood pressure and family health history.

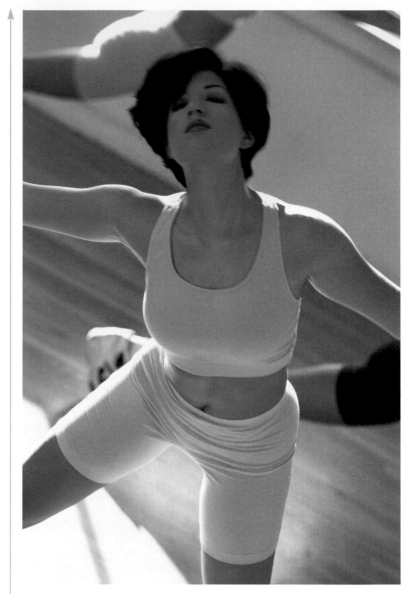

People who become even moderately active can cut their risk of heart disease by as much as half. If you already have heart disease, exercise can lower your risk of heart attack and stroke.

in your way. Maybe you often have to grab lunch on the run—and the only place to stop is a fast-food joint. Maybe you're doing fine until you dine out, and then you eat a lot more than you should. For each obstacle, think of a way around it—packing a lunch, for instance, or dividing that gigantic plate of pasta at your favorite restaurant in half and having the waiter put it in a doggie bag even before you start eating.

4. Action. You've already turned intent into action. For almost anyone who tries to make a lifestyle change, obstacles can appear, sometimes out of nowhere. Remind yourself that a small lapse doesn't mean you've fallen apart. Plan ahead with strategies for times when you may find it hard to stick with your goals (around the holidays, for instance).

5. Maintenance. If you've already reached Stage Five, congratulations! You're well on your way to a heart-healthy life. At this stage, it's important to remind yourself of the many benefits you're reaping and to stick with the program. In *Heart Healthy for Life* we'll give you tips on how to make your new habits last a lifetime.

Never too late ... or too early

Younger adults tend to think they're invincible. The threat of problems like cancer or heart disease seems so distant that these people rarely take the risk seriously. On the other hand, older individuals sometimes think it's too late to make meaningful changes because the damage is already done.

Both groups are dead wrong. When researchers perform autopsies on people as young as 25, they frequently find signs of fatty streaks in blood vessel walls—evidence that the process of atherosclerosis has already begun. Nearly 15 percent of all kids in the United States have elevated cholesterol levels. True, some of them suffer from familial hypercholesterolemia, an inherited condition that causes abnormally high cholesterol. But most have high cholesterol simply because they eat too much saturated fat. It's never too early, in other words, to start taking care of your heart.

Or too late. There's plenty of evidence that older folks who make heart-healthy changes reap the benefits in spades. For instance, University of California heart expert Dean Ornish, M.D., has shown that people with advanced heart disease can improve the health of their arteries through a rigorous program of diet and exercise along with stress-reduction techniques. And researchers at the Cooper Institute for Aerobics Research in Dallas, Texas, found that older men who exercised and improved their overall fitness reduced their risk of dying over the five-year study period by 44 percent. Even longtime smokers can reduce the heart-related damage caused by cigarettes if they quit today.

There's no better time than right now, in other words, to take the first step toward a healthier heart. And *Heart Healthy for Life* will show you how.

Younger adults tend to think they're invincible. On the other hand, older individuals sometimes think it's too late to make meaningful changes.

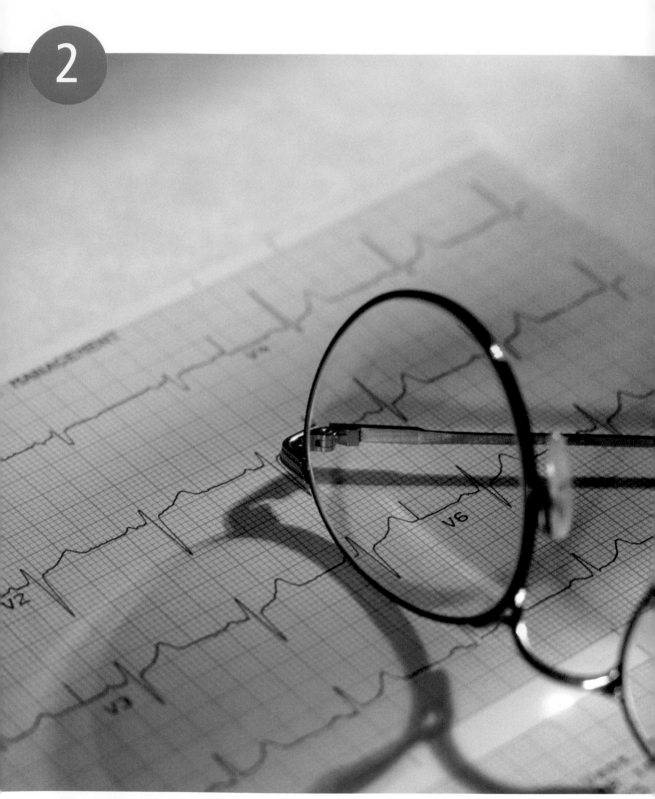

Assessing Your Risk

Fifty years ago, the cause of most heart attacks was a mystery. No one knew why they happened at all—let alone why they happened to some people and not others. Today, researchers are clued in to many of the factors that put people in the path of danger. Knowing exactly how you stack up in these areas will help you and your doctor target a powerful prevention strategy tailored to your risk profile.

Some points against you, like a family history of heart disease, you simply have to swallow. But by disarming the hazards under your control, like high blood pressure or high cholesterol, you can slash your risk for a heart attack or stroke. If you've already had one, you can go a long way toward avoiding another.

An International Detective Story

When researchers first began to unravel the mystery of heart disease, they began with one tantalizing clue: the odd fact that the risk for heart attacks varied dramatically in different parts of the world. In Finland and the United States, for instance, heart disease topped the list of leading causes of death. In other places, like Greece, it was exceedingly rare.

In a now famous investigation called the Seven Countries Study, scientists back in the 1950s set out to discover why. They compared thousands of people in Japan, the United States, Greece, Italy, Finland, the former Yugoslavia, and the Netherlands, using blood tests and survey questionnaires. One of their first discoveries was that cholesterol levels in the blood also varied widely in different parts of the world. What's more, there seemed to be a close connection between these levels and the risk for heart attacks. The higher a person's cholesterol, the greater the danger.

Since then, researchers have identified a host of other factors that increase a person's likelihood of developing heart disease. Some are aspects of ourselves we can't alter, such as our age, gender, or family health history. Fortunately, many more are things we can change. These include certain medical conditions (for instance, diabetes and high blood pressure) that if left untreated can damage arteries or weaken the heart. They also include

"By disarming the hazards under your control, like high blood pressure or high cholesterol, you can slash your risk for a heart attack or stroke."

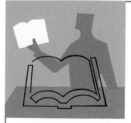

TERMS TO KNOW

BODY MASS INDEX (BMI) A scale used to measure body mass. Your body mass index is your body weight in pounds divided by your height in inches squared

CONGESTIVE HEART FAILURE A condition that occurs when the heart can no longer efficiently pump blood around the body, leading to a buildup of fluid in the lungs and body tissues

DIASTOLIC The bottom number of a blood pressure reading. Diastolic blood pressure is the lowest pressure that occurs when the heart relaxes between beats

HDL High-density lipoprotein, a beneficial component of cholesterol that promotes the breakdown and removal of artery-clogging cholesterol

HYPERCHOLESTEROLEMIA An inherited form of high cholesterol that significantly increases heart disease risk

HYPERTENSION High blood pressure

LDL Low-density lipoprotein, the dangerous component of cholesterol that can gather on the inside of blood vessels, forming deposits that block blood flow

SYSTOLIC The top number of a blood pressure reading. Systolic blood pressure is the highest pressure that occurs when the heart contracts with each heartbeat

TRIGLYCERIDES Fat particles in the blood, which can increase cardiovascular disease risk when they occur at high levels

lifestyle factors, such as diet and exercise, over which we have absolute control.

A word about risk

Having one or more risk factors for heart disease doesn't mean you're doomed to have a heart attack. Think seat belts. Driving without a seat belt dramatically increases your chances of being severely injured or dying in a crash. Of course, some people who don't use seat belts will never be in an accident, and some who do may be hurt or killed in a car. But overall, the risks are much greater if you don't wear seat belts than if you do.

The same goes for heart disease. Just as not wearing a seat belt increases your chances of being injured in an accident, elevated cholesterol or high blood pressure jacks up your odds for having heart problems down the road. Eliminating or lessening such a risk can dramatically lower the hazard.

What if you don't have any risk factors? Are you safe from ever having a heart attack? Not entirely. For, while you're significantly less likely to develop heart disease, some heart attacks occur out of the blue, in the absence of any known risk factors. Why remains a mystsery.

But one thing is clear: Adding more exercise to your life, helping yourself to more heart-protective foods, and learning to put stress in its place are smart moves even if you aren't in any imminent danger. Think of them as an insurance policy against heart problems and all kinds of other illnesses, including diabetes and many cancers.

Risk Factors You Can't Change

It may seem odd to worry about things you can't change. But recognizing your risk factors is essential to knowing your overall probability of developing heart disease in the next 10 years. Plus, it creates real incentive to take charge of what you can change. Here are the main risks you may be stuck with.

1. Inherited risk. If heart disease runs in your family—especially heart attacks that occur before the age of 50 for men and 55 for women—you're likely to be at increased risk. The most significant threat is associated with an inherited condition called familial hypercholesterolemia, which causes dangerously high cholesterol levels (350 mg/dL, or 350 milligrams per deciliter of blood). A tendency toward high blood pressure, obesity, or diabetes can also be inherited.

Does a family history of early heart disease mean you're fated to have it, too? Not at all. But knowing your family history will help you and your doctor target the wisest prevention strategy. If you have hypercholesterolemia, for instance, your doctor is likely to recommend dietary changes and/or medications to bring your cholesterol level down and keep it down.

2. Gender. More men than women develop cardiovascular disease. Men also develop it about a decade earlier than women do. Researchers don't know exactly why premenopausal women are protected, although estrogen may play a role. After menopause, as

WHITE COAT HYPERTENSION

Blood pressure typically rises when people are nervous or under stress. Ironically, one place that often causes stress—and raises blood pressure—is a doctor's office. Researchers call this phenomenon white coat hypertension, referring to the white coat doctors typically wear. If your blood pressure registers high, your doctor may recommend taking a few readings on your own, either at home or at blood pressure stations found in some drugstores or supermarkets.

To measure your pressure at home, you'll need a device called a sphygmomanometer (pronounced SFIG-mo-mah-NOM-uh-tur), which uses the arm cuff that you're familiar with. Your doctor will explain when and how to use it.

estrogen levels decline, a woman's risk begins to rise. As men and women reach their 60s and 70s, the gender gap narrows. In the end, 47 percent of all fatal heart attacks occur in women.

3. Age. Risk increases with age. Half of all heart attacks in the United States occur in people over 65. That doesn't mean that cardiovascular disease is an inevitable part of aging, however. In some parts of the world, it remains far less common at any age than it is in the United States. Why? A lifetime of healthful eating and plenty of physical activity can protect most people throughout their lives.

Risk Factors You Can Change

The risk factors you can change far outnumber those you can't. That's terrific news. It means that even if you have a family history of heart disease you can make a huge dent in your inherited risk. Factors you can change come in two categories: medical conditions that contribute to heart disease and habits that affect your heart.

Medical conditions

1. High blood pressure.

To supply oxygen and nutrients to every part of the body, your heart must pump with enough force, or pressure, to keep blood moving. When blood flow becomes restricted in the smaller branches of the arteries, the pressure has to be increased in order to push the blood through. (The same thing happens when you put your finger over the end of a garden hose. As you restrict the flow of water, the pressure increases.) The result is high blood pressure, also known as hypertension. This condition puts strain on the blood ves-

Key Finding

Even blood pressure in the high-normal range (130-139/85-89) may be too high, according to a 2001 report from researchers involved in the Framingham Heart Study. Comparing people with optimal blood pressure (under 120/80), those with slightly elevated numbers were found to be two times more likely to develop cardiovascular disease. Blood pressure in the high-normal range was found to be particularly dangerous for women, the study found.

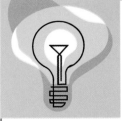

ASK THE EXPERT

"How can some cholesterol be good and some bad?"

James Cleeman, M.D., director of the National Cholesterol Education Program:

"The difference between good and bad cholesterol is really the difference in the direction cholesterol is traveling in the blood: into the tissues of the body, where it can accumulate inside artery walls, or back to the liver, where it is eliminated.

First, a word about cholesterol. All cholesterol in the blood takes the form of small packets called lipoproteins, made up of fat (also called lipids) and protein. Just as oil and water don't mix, fat and blood don't mix. So lipoproteins are constructed with the fat on the inside and the protein molecules on the outside, allowing them to travel easily through the blood.

Low-density lipoprotein, or LDL (the so-called bad cholesterol), is cholesterol on its way into the tissues of the body, including artery walls. Too much of it can build up to create plaques on the lining of blood vessels. Blood clots can attach themselves to these plaques, cutting off blood flow and causing a heart attack. In contrast, high-density lipoprotein, or HDL (the so-called good cholesterol), is cholesterol being carried away from the tissues to the liver for disposal.

It makes good sense, of course, to want to keep your levels of LDL low and your HDL high. In fact, we have very solid evidence that lowering your LDL levels will reduce heart attack risk. We have less evidence that raising HDL levels will bring down the danger, although most researchers are pretty sure it will. As it happens, we're much better at lowering LDL—through dietary changes or medication—than we are at raising HDL.

There are certainly ways to bring HDL numbers up—by increasing physical activity, for instance, and quitting smoking—and this is very important to heart health. But reducing LDL levels should be the prime focus of our efforts."

sels and on the heart. If left untreated, it can inflate your odds of developing coronary artery disease by as much as threefold and your chances of having a stroke by sevenfold.

These numbers are all the more worrisome because as many as 50 million Americans suffer from high blood pressure. And nearly one in three doesn't even know he or she has it. High blood pressure is sometimes called a silent killer because it has no symptoms. The only way to diagnose it is to have your blood pressure tested. If your numbers are in the red zone (see page 28), there are plenty of ways to bring them down.

WHAT THE NUMBERS MEAN

BLOOD PRESSURE

Blood pressure is measured in millimeters of mercury, or mmHg. It includes two numbers, usually written as a fraction. The top number represents systolic blood pressure, or the highest pressure that occurs when your heart is contracting. The bottom number represents diastolic blood pressure, or the lowest pressure that occurs when your heart is relaxing and filling with blood.

The average healthy person has a blood pressure of 120/70. A reading of 140/90 is considered borderline high blood pressure. Anything above 150/100 is considered high blood pressure.

CHOLESTEROL

Until recently, most blood tests for cholesterol measured only total cholesterol. Now researchers know that one form of the substance, called low-density lipoprotein, or LDL, is especially harmful to arteries. Another form, called high-density lipoprotein, or HDL, actually keeps arteries clear by removing the bad form. By comparing levels of HDL and LDL, doctors get a fairly reliable picture of your risk for heart disease. Your cholesterol screening results can also help your doctor advise you on the best way to improve your cholesterol profile and lower your heart disease risk. Experts from the National Cholesterol Education Program recently released these new guidelines for target cholesterol levels.

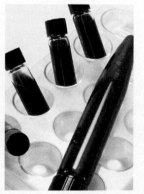

If you're healthy
- Total cholesterol: less than 200 mg/dL
- HDL cholesterol: more than 40 mg/dL
- LDL cholesterol: less than 130 mg/dL

If you have coronary artery disease
- Total cholesterol: less than 200 mg/dL
- HDL cholesterol: more than 40 mg/dL
- LDL cholesterol: less than 100 mg/dL

TRIGLYCERIDES

Cholesterol tests also typically measure the level of triglyceride, the other major fat, in the blood. Many studies have shown a strong connection between elevated triglyceride levels and increased risk of heart disease—although the link isn't as strong as that for cholesterol or high blood pressure. One reason is that triglyceride levels vary widely from person to person. Men tend to have higher levels than women. What's more, there is no evidence that high levels actually cause heart disease (unlike cholesterol, which plays a key role). Still, your doctor may want to know your levels in order to fine-tune your prescription for lowering your heart attack risk.

Triglyceride levels below 200 mg/dL are considered healthy; a reading higher than 200 indicates increased risk. Fortunately, the same lifestyle changes that can lower your cholesterol will also improve your triglyceride numbers. Losing weight may be especially important, since elevated triglycerides are associated with obesity.

2. High cholesterol. The higher your total cholesterol, the greater your danger. In the Framingham Heart Study, researchers found that people with a total cholesterol of 300 mg/dL were twice as likely to develop heart disease as people with numbers around 150 mg/dL. In another, more recent study, the Multiple Risk Factor Intervention Trial, high cholesterol looked even more perilous. Of the 360,000 men studied, those with total cholesterol above 300 mg/dL were four times more likely to die of heart disease during the study than men with numbers below 180 mg/dL.

What's wrong with having too much cholesterol? The form of the waxy substance known as low-density lipoprotein, or LDL cholesterol, can build up inside artery walls, causing accumulations called plaques. These plaques lead to atherosclerosis (hardening of the arteries) and may eventually cause heart attacks or strokes. There are many ways to bring down high LDL cholesterol, from cutting back on saturated fat and eating more fruit and vegetables to taking one of the new generation of cholesterol-lowering medications.

LDL isn't the whole story. Scientists now know that high density lipoprotein, or HDL, is also important. HDL helps remove damaging cholesterol from the blood. So the higher your level of this form of cholesterol, the lower your danger of clogged arteries—and heart attacks. The National Cholesterol Education Program recently revised upward its recommendation for a healthy HDL level, from 35 mg/dL to 40 mg/dL. The reason: Studies show that people with levels below 40 mg/dL have a higher than average risk of developing coronary artery disease. Those with levels above 60 mg/dL are significantly less likely to experience heart problems.

3. Diabetes. Diabetes impairs the body's ability to process sugar for energy. Your body normally converts some of the food you eat into glucose, a type of sugar. The hormone called insulin allows glucose to enter cells, where it is used for energy. Two forms of diabetes can disrupt this finely calibrated system. Type I diabetes occurs when the pancreas fails to produce enough insulin to process glucose. Type II diabetes, also called adult-onset diabetes, occurs when cells stop responding normally to insulin. If you have either one, your risk of cardiovascular disease is roughly twice that of the general population. Fortunately, for most people, medications and lifestyle changes can keep diabetes from threatening your heart or causing a stroke.

FAST FACT

As many as five to seven million Americans with diabetes don't know they have the condition, which can at least double the risk for heart disease.

Lifestyle factors that increase risk

One of the biggest breakthroughs of modern medicine has nothing to do with fancy tests or high-tech procedures. It's the discovery that many chronic diseases, including cardiovascular disease, are caused in large part by the way we live. The main lifestyle factors that influence heart disease risk include smoking, being overweight, being sedentary, and eating a poor diet.

1. Smoking. Cigarette smoke delivers hundreds of toxic substances and gases into your lungs and bloodstream. Some of these directly harm the heart. Nicotine increases blood pressure and heart rate. Carbon monoxide—the same gas your car's tailpipe spews—reduces the amount of oxygen your blood can carry, forcing your heart to work harder than normal. It also robs heart muscle of the blood and oxygen it needs to function properly.

Every year, more than 430,000 people die as a result of smoking—one-third of them from cardiovascular disease. Smoking increases your risk of atherosclerosis by 50 percent and speeds up the damage to your arteries by 10 years. The earlier you begin smoking and the more cigarettes you light up, the greater the danger. Smoke a pack a day, and your risk of cardiovascular disease is at least twice as high as that of a nonsmoker. Smoke two or more packs, and it climbs to threefold. If you've tried to quit without success, it's time to try again. New smoking cessation aids such as nicotine patches have been shown to double your odds of succeeding.

So-called secondhand smoke isn't as dangerous as directly inhaled smoke, but it does increase your risk. In fact, it is thought to be directly responsible for more than 50,000 deaths from cardiovascular disease each year.

2. Being overweight. The nation's weight problem is bad and getting worse. Today, 30 percent of Americans are overweight. Another 25 percent are obese, or severely overweight. In fact, obesity has increased 91 percent in the past decade. More than half of

Key Finding

As dangerous as smoking is for men, it may be even more hazardous for women. Smoking lowers the level of estrogen in a woman's body. That's worrisome, since many experts believe estrogen protects women from cardiovascular disease prior to menopause. Women who smoke and use oral contraceptives, especially women over age 35, have higher rates of heart disease than nonsmokers. Although no one knows exactly why, smoking in combination with using oral contraceptives seems to increase blood pressure and cholesterol levels.

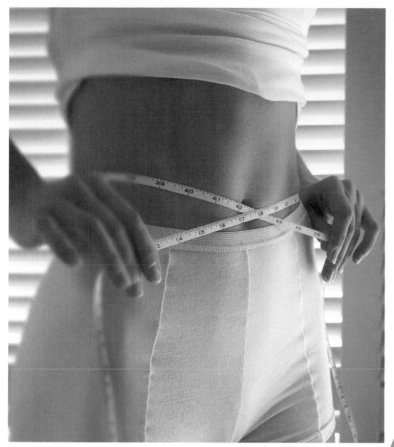

Losing just 4 percent of your body weight can significantly lower your total cholesterol.

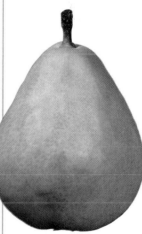

us, in other words, weigh more than we should. And all that excess weight adds to heart disease risk. Why? Even body fat needs oxygen and nutrients, which is supplied by blood. More fat requires more blood, which leads to high blood pressure. Being overweight also increases the possibility of diabetes. And the simple fact that your body is forced to carry more weight than it was built for strains your heart, adding to the risk of congestive heart failure in people with cardiovascular disease.

3. Being sedentary. What's wrong with doing nothing? Plenty. Being sedentary increases the risk of diabetes and high blood pressure. Couch potatoes are also more likely to be overweight. And when people aren't active, their heart muscles get out of shape, just like the rest of their muscles. That can make the heart more vulnerable to damage. Studies show that being sedentary doubles your risk of suffering a heart attack.

Yet more than 6 out of 10 of us don't get the recommended dose of exercise (at least 30 minutes of activities like brisk walking

FAST FACT

Are you shaped more like an apple or a pear? If your body fat is distributed mostly around your stomach (instead of your buttocks, hips, and thighs), you're at greater risk for heart disease.

most days of the week). One out of 4 reports doing no physical activity at all. If you spend most of your time sitting, it's high time to get your heart pumping.

Deadly combinations

It's obvious that the more risk factors you have, the greater your odds of developing heart disease or, if you already have it, of suffering a heart attack or stroke. But some factors, when added together, create a combined risk that's greater than you'd expect. Having high cholesterol and smoking, for example, seems to be a particularly menacing combination.

Luckily, there's an up side. By erasing just one risk factor—say, smoking—you will take some of the sting out of other dangers, such as high cholesterol. Eliminate two risk factors and you may gain more than double the benefits for your efforts.

> "Having high cholesterol and smoking seems to be a particularly menacing combination."

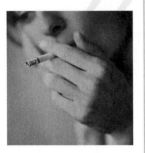

Beating the Big Three

In the years since researchers fingered high blood pressure, high cholesterol, and smoking as the principal enemies of the heart, we've made big strides in bringing them to justice.

- The prevalence of high blood pressure in the United States has declined 40 percent.
- The number of Americans with dangerously high cholesterol has fallen 28 percent.
- The percentage of Americans who smoke has dropped from 33 percent to 25 percent.

But plenty of people remain at risk. Experts from the National Cholesterol Education Program recently warned, for instance, that as many as 53 million Americans have dangerously high cholesterol levels. Only half of the estimated 50 million people in the United States with high blood pressure are being treated with medication. And some 49 million Americans continue to smoke. On top of all this, we're gaining more weight and getting less exercise.

Are we doomed? Certainly not. Making even small inroads against key risk factors, it turns out, can make a big difference. Consider elevated cholesterol. For every one percent drop in total cholesterol, you get a two to three percent reduction in heart disease risk. That's an impressive return on investment. In fact, as long as your level isn't sky-high, there's a good chance you can

WHAT'S YOUR RISK?

By answering a few simple questions, you can get a good idea of your own risk of developing heart disease over the next 10 years. To take this quiz, you'll need to know your blood pressure, total cholesterol, and body mass index (see page 131). This test is not for people who have already been diagnosed with cardiovascular disease. Nor does it take the place of a medical examination and doctor's advice. To calculate your risk, add the numbers beside the boxes you've checked.

I am
❥ Male under 40 1
❥ Male 40 or older 2
❥ Female and have not gone
   through menopause 1
❥ Female and have gone
   through menopause 2

My BMI is
❥ 19 to 24 0
❥ 25 to 29. 1
❥ 30 or higher. 2

I exercise
❥ More than 30 minutes
   most days of the week 0
❥ Up to 30 minutes most
   days of the week 1
❥ Very little 2

My total cholesterol is
❥ 200 mg/dL or below. 0
❥ 200 to 240 mg/dL. 1
❥ Above 240 mg/dL. 2

My blood pressure is
❥ Below 140/90. 0
❥ Between 140/90 and 160/90 1
❥ Above 160/90 2

My smoking history is
❥ Never smoked 0
❥ Quit more than three years ago 1
❥ Don't smoke but
   live with people
   who do 2
❥ Quit less than
   three years ago. 2
❥ Currently smoke. 3

I have high blood sugar
levels or diabetes
❥ No 0
❥ Yes 2

My family history is
❥ No known family history
   of early heart attacks 0
❥ Mother or sister who had a
   heart attack before age 65. 2
❥ Father or brother who had a
   heart attack before age 55. 2

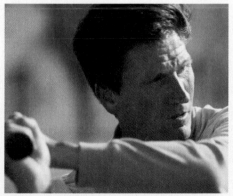

A score of **0 to 4** indicates very low risk of developing heart disease.

A score of **5 to 8** indicates moderate risk of developing heart disease.

A score of **9 to 17** indicates high risk of developing heart disease.

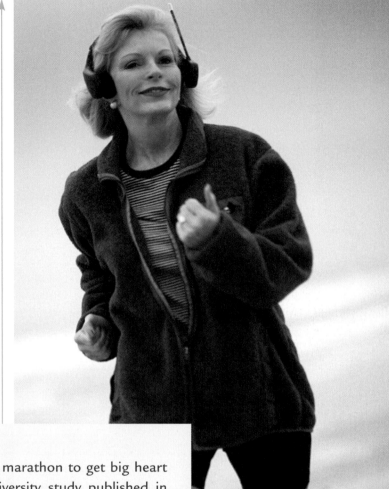

Key Finding

You don't have to run a marathon to get big heart benefits. A Harvard University study published in 2001 showed that women who walked just one hour a week lowered their risk of heart disease by 14 percent. Those who hit the pavement for 1.5 hours a week reduced their risk by 51 percent compared with women who rarely walk. Time spent walking, the researchers found, was more important in reducing heart disease risk than walking pace.

bring it into the safe zone by making a few lifestyle adjustments. What'll it take? Smarter eating, for starters. Follow the American Heart Association's recommended diet, which advises consuming no more than 30 percent of calories from fat and only 10 percent from saturated fats and hydrogenated oils, and if you're like most people, you can bring your LDL cholesterol level down by 15 percent. Adding a few helpings of high-fiber foods can bring the numbers down, too. In findings published in 2001, University of Toronto researcher David Jenkins, Ph.D., showed that a diet that includes more than one-third of its

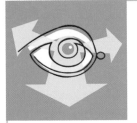

LOOKING AHEAD
New clues to heart disease risk

Although major factors like high blood pressure and elevated cholesterol alert doctors to patients at increased danger for heart disease, they don't identify everyone. Significant numbers of people with no known risk factors have heart attacks. Researchers continue to search for the missing links. So far, several new clues have been identified that may help doctors pinpoint your risk.

Homocysteine High blood levels of this amino acid have been linked to increased risk of heart disease. Homocysteine is believed to damage cells that line the coronary arteries. Fortunately folate, a form of B vitamin, keeps levels in check. That's why experts say it's important to get 400 micrograms of folate every day. Now that breads and cereals are fortified with the nutrient, most Americans get enough in their diets. A daily multivitamin offers added insurance. Some researchers believe folate supplementation may explain the decrease in heart disease that has occurred over the past few decades.

Lipoprotein(a) Although low-density lipoproteins, or LDL (the "bad" cholesterol), are infamous for clogging blood vessels, other lipoproteins may also spell trouble. One currently under investigation, known as Lp(a), has been linked to higher risk of early heart disease. Lp(a) may prevent clots from being dissolved, increasing the danger of a blockage of blood flow to the heart.

Infectious germs Experts have uncovered evidence that infectious germs may damage blood vessel walls, increasing the risk of atherosclerosis and blood clots. Culprits include cytomegalovirus, chlamydia, and H. pylori. A study published in 2001 looked at 1,018 patients with coronary artery disease. The more germs they tested positive for, the greater their chances of dying from their disease.

C-reactive protein Inflammation, a natural reaction to injury or infection, may fast-forward the process of atherosclerosis. Scientists have identified a substance called C-reactive protein that serves as a marker for inflammation. In one recent study, men with high levels of the protein had a threefold higher risk for heart attack. Some cardiologists now test for C-reactive protein in patients with cardiovascular disease, although others question the value of the results.

HPA-2 Met A common gene variation dubbed HPA-2 Met makes blood stickier and more likely to clot, according to a 2001 study by scientists in Finland. Men with this trait were found to have double the risk of sudden cardiac death. The gene may also predispose men to coronary thrombosis, or a blood clot in the heart. There is currently no screening test for HPA-2 Met. If anyone in your family has died of premature cardiac arrest, it's important to be screened for other known risk factors, such as high blood pressure and elevated cholesterol. Eventually, researchers believe that genetic tests will play a key role in identifying people at increased heart disease risk.

calories from fruit, vegetables, and nuts (yes, nuts!) can lower LDL cholesterol by a whopping 33 percent.

Get moving, and you'll coax those numbers down even farther. When volunteers in a recent Stanford University study switched to a low-fat diet, their LDL levels fell by 7 to 11 percent. When they added exercise—walking or jogging 10 miles a week—the numbers tumbled almost twice as far. The most important benefit of exercise is its ability to boost HDL, the good cholesterol. In another Stanford study, volunteers who walked or jogged 9 miles a week saw their HDL levels climb 13 percent. Add it all up, and what have you got? With lifestyle changes alone, research shows, most individuals can bring elevated cholesterol levels down 20 to 30 percent. That's enough to keep many people with high cholesterol from needing cholesterol-lowering drugs. Even for those who do need medication, getting heart smart can help reduce the dose.

HOT TOPIC
Syndrome X: The Fearful Foursome

Experts have long known that the more risk factors a person has, the greater the danger of heart disease. But Gerald Reaven, M.D., a researcher at Stanford University School of Medicine, believes that one distinct quartet of factors may be especially dangerous. The combination includes high blood pressure, high triglycerides, low HDL (the so-called good cholesterol), and obesity. Together, these four factors, dubbed metabolic syndrome, or Syndrome X, dramatically increase a person's chances of developing coronary artery disease.

At the core of Syndrome X is insulin resistance, a condition in which when cells don't respond to insulin normally. To compensate, the body churns out extra insulin in order to bring the amount of blood sugar, or glucose, in the bloodstream under control by moving it into cells. This extra insulin may in turn damage the interior lining of blood vessels, increasing the threat of heart attack. According to the long-running Quebec Cardiovascular Study, every 30 percent increase in insulin is associated with a 70 percent increase in the risk of heart disease over a period of five years.

If you have the four risk factors that make up the syndrome, it may be particularly important for your doctor to monitor your blood glucose levels, cholesterol levels, and blood pressure. Weight loss and exercise are especially key.

For people with insulin resistance, Dr. Reaven recommends against the low-fat, high-carbohydrate diet espoused by the American Heart Association, since people with insulin resistance have to secrete more insulin in order to process carbohydrates. High-protein diets also increase insulin secretion. But dietary fat has no effect on insulin levels. Therefore, Dr. Reaven advises a relatively high-fat diet made up of 40 percent fats (30 to 35 percent heart-healthy unsaturated fats), 45 percent carbohydrates, and 15 percent protein.

Will it work for you?

Diet and exercise efforts don't have the same effect on everyone. Some people can make a small change and see a big payoff. Others can work hard and see only a small improvement. Take cholesterol. Researchers have found that about 20 percent of adults are "nonresponders"—that is, their cholesterol levels won't budge even on the best diet and exercise regimen. Another 20 percent, called hyperresponders, will never have to worry about their cholesterol levels no matter what they eat.

Unfair? Sure. But remember: Even if you're among those who can't lower cholesterol levels without medication, a healthier diet and plenty of physical activity have many other health benefits.

5 Things You Can Do Today to Lower Your Risk

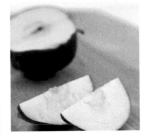

1

Eat one extra serving of fruit and one extra serving of vegetables.

2

Take a multivitamin.

3

Go for a walk. How fast you walk isn't that important. Just aim to walk for at least 30 minutes (depending on your current level of fitness).

4

If you don't know your cholesterol levels, make an appointment to be tested.

5

Starting today, if you smoke, smoke one less cigarette a day until you're ready to quit.

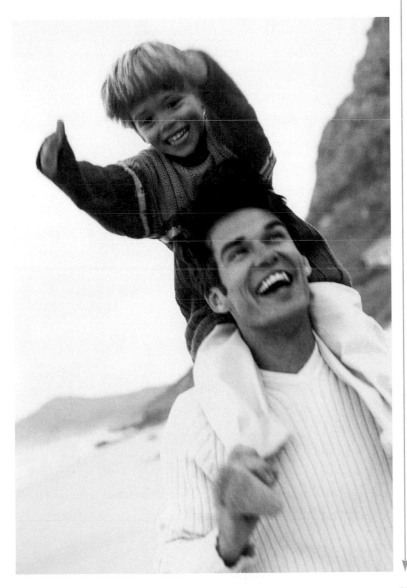

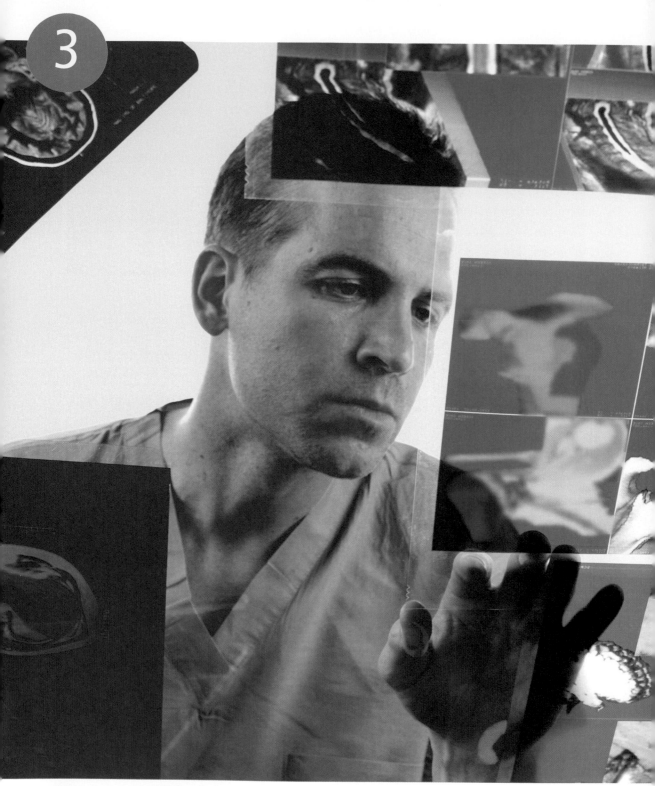

Spotting Trouble

Too many people don't know they have heart disease until their first heart attack—more than half of which prove fatal. Many of those deaths could be prevented. Today, sophisticated new tests can help your doctor detect signs of trouble earlier and more accurately than ever before.

Using advanced imaging techniques, for instance, physicians can create a detailed map of your heart and arteries, pinpointing cholesterol buildup or damage to heart muscle without ever picking up a scalpel. They can then use this information to take targeted action that could save your life.

Tricky Business

Even with the latest advances, however, diagnosing heart disease can be difficult. One reason is that many different types of heart problems can arise. Some affect the valves of the heart. Others interfere with blood flow into the heart. Still others may be the result of damage to blood vessels elsewhere in the body.

Complicating matters, more than one problem may show up in the same patient. For example, someone with atherosclerosis may develop both coronary artery disease (affecting blood flow to the heart) and carotid artery disease (affecting blood flow to the brain). And a heart attack can lead to congestive heart failure, which occurs when damage to the heart interferes with its ability to pump blood efficiently everywhere that it's needed.

Another factor is that coronary artery disease, the leading cause of heart attacks, occurs slowly, usually over the course of many years. Atherosclerosis begins when substances such as cholesterol are deposited in fatty streaks on the arteries' inner lining. Researchers have found early signs of this condition in people as young as 25. As these fatty deposits accumulate, other substances can adhere to them, including fibrous tissue, various blood components, and calcium. These harden into scablike lesions called plaques, which begin to obstruct blood flow. For reasons that are only beginning to be understood, an area of plaque can break loose, plugging up the artery entirely. Alternatively, a blood clot can form on top of a plaque, cutting off blood supply to the heart and causing a heart attack.

Coronary artery disease, the leading cause of heart attacks, occurs slowly, usually over the course of many years.

Most people don't know they have a problem until their coronary arteries become so obstructed that blood flow becomes severely restricted. This can cause symptoms such as chest tightness or shortness of breath. Or, if a blood clot abruptly closes off a constricted artery, it can trigger a heart attack.

Early warning signs

The majority of heart attacks don't have to happen. Once coronary artery disease is diagnosed, its progress can be slowed, halted, or even reversed through effective treatment and lifestyle changes, such as a healthier diet and more physical activity. An important part of defending your heart is being aware of early symptoms—especially if you know you are at elevated risk of heart disease. Not everyone experiences coronary artery disease in the same way, but here are a few common warning signs.

IS IT ANGINA?

How do you know if the pain in your chest is angina? It's not always easy even for doctors to recognize angina and distinguish it from other kinds of chest pain. Angina is usually experienced as pressure or squeezing in the middle of the chest behind the breastbone. The pressure, sometimes described as heavy, crushing, or like a vise, may radiate up into the throat or jaw or up into the left shoulder and down the left arm. Angina is usually worse in cold weather, during physical activities, following a meal, or after emotional stress.

The symptom of chest pressure or shortness of breath can have other causes, of course. Shortness of breath can be trig-

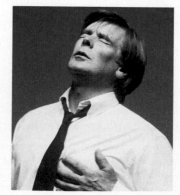

gered by lung-related illnesses, such as bronchitis or emphysema. Chest pain can be caused by viral infections, strained muscles, even plain old indigestion. Still, symptoms like these shouldn't be taken lightly. If you have them, see your doctor. If he believes there is cause for concern, he may order one or more tests, such as an electrocardiogram, designed to diagnose specific heart problems.

If you experience chest pain that doesn't subside within a few minutes—especially if you know you are at high risk for coronary artery disease—chew an aspirin and get someone to drive you to an emergency room immediately, or call 911 for an ambulance.

Ischemia: blood flow reduces to a trickle. The first sign of serious trouble from atherosclerosis is ischemia, which simply means decreased blood flow. "Myocardial ischemia" refers to reduced flow of blood through the coronary arteries that feed the heart. Some patients with myocardial ischemia have symptoms that tip off doctors that the heart is beginning to be robbed of oxygen and nutrients, such as a tightness in the chest or weakness when they exert themselves.

Angina: a pain in the chest. As the arteries that supply the heart become more and more obstructed, some people experience a form of chest pain called angina. It often shows up first when they are under physical or emotional stress—shoveling snow, for instance, or arguing with a spouse. Angina triggered by exercise, sometimes called exertional angina, usually subsides when people stop what they're doing and rest. As the artery blockages become worse, however, angina may happen when people are doing nothing more strenuous than sitting still or even sleeping.

Angina that occurs at rest usually indicates more serious ischemia. Constricted arteries can no longer supply even the minimal amount of oxygenated blood the heart needs. When angina enters this phase, it is sometimes called unstable angina. The reason: The blood supply to the heart has become so restricted that a heart attack can occur at almost any time.

Heart attack: when the damage turns deadly

Unfortunately, some patients never experience pain in their chest until the arteries that serve the heart become completely obstructed, cutting off blood flow to parts of the heart and causing a heart attack. This can happen when one of the scablike plaques breaks free from the artery wall and plugs up a narrowed section of the

Angina triggered by exercise, sometimes called exertional angina, usually subsides when people stop what they're doing and rest.

artery. It can also result when a blood clot forms in arteries already constricted by atherosclerosis. If the blood supply is cut off long enough—around 30 minutes—heart muscle cells begin to die.

The American Heart Association has identified three common warning signals of a heart attack. They are:

- Uncomfortable pressure, fullness, squeezing or pain in the center of your chest lasting more than a few minutes. (This feeling of pressure isn't necessarily located right over the heart. It can occur anywhere in the chest.)
- Pain spreading to the shoulders, neck, or arms.
- Lightheadedness, fainting, sweating, nausea, or shortness of breath, usually accompanied by discomfort in your chest.

Other, less common symptoms include stomach or abdominal pain, difficulty breathing, unexplained anxiety or fatigue, and palpitations or cold sweats. Keep in mind: Not all of them occur in every heart attack. And some come and go.

Unfortunately, of the estimated 1.2 million people who have heart attacks every year, only about 950,000 make it to an emergency room. The rest die before they can get lifesaving care. If you think you may be having a heart attack, call 911 and then take an aspirin, either chewing it or putting it under your tongue to speed its absorption into the bloodstream, instead of simply swallowing it. Aspirin helps thin the blood and keep it flowing.

Key Finding

More than 600 people die from cardiac arrest outside of hospitals every day. Many more would survive, experts say, if more defibrillators were available in public places like airports, shopping malls, train stations, and office buildings—and if more people were trained in how to use them. Automatic external defibrillators, or AEDs, are devices used by emergency medical technicians to "shock" the heart of someone in cardiac arrest into beating normally again. When researchers placed AEDs in casinos in Las Vegas and trained security guards in their use, survival rates for people suffering heart attacks in America's gambling capital soared.

Heart failure: weak but still beating

A heart attack and heart failure may sound like the same thing, but they represent very different conditions. A heart attack occurs when a blockage in one of the coronary arteries suddenly cuts off blood supply to the heart, causing serious damage to heart muscles. Heart failure, in contrast, typically develops slowly as the heart muscle grows weaker and weaker, becoming less efficient at pumping blood.

A CLOSER LOOK AT LIPIDS

Many university hospitals and major medical centers now offer lipid clinics. These state-of-the-art facilities look beyond standard cholesterol tests at a variety of more subtle clues to heart attack risk.

The reason: Standard risk factors account for only about half of all cases of coronary artery disease. Fifty percent of all people who develop heart problems, in other words, don't have the usual early warning signs of high blood pressure or elevated cholesterol. At lipid clinics, doctors and researchers use more sophisticated blood tests to try to spot hidden danger signs.

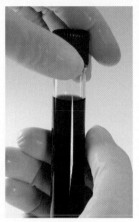

Patients are typically referred to a lipid clinic after they've been diagnosed with atherosclerosis or angina or after they've suffered a heart attack. Experts say it's also a good idea to visit a lipid clinic if you have a strong family history of early heart attacks.

One goal of these clinics is to unravel the mystery of why a person with no known risk factors suddenly develops heart disease. "We may see a patient whose total HDL levels look fine, but when we look more closely at the HDL, we discover defects that may get in the way of its transporting cholesterol out of the body" says Mary Malloy, M.D., who heads up the lipid clinic at the University of California at San Francisco (UCSF). Researchers may also find defects in LDL particles that prevent them from being cleared from the bloodstream normally.

The tests offered at lipid clinics can help doctors choose the best treatment. Patients who have a certain defect in their LDL may be less sensitive to cholesterol-lowering statin drugs, for instance. In that case, they may fare better on niacin, which improves cholesterol status by raising HDL. Patients who are discovered to have high blood levels of cardiac C-reactive protein, which indicates inflammation, may be treated with an antibiotic. Chronic inflammation can injure the lining of artery walls, making them more susceptible to cholesterol buildup.

Another goal of many lipid clinics is to advance the science of detecting heart disease risk. At UCSF's lipid clinic, researchers are screening blood from 20,000 patients with atherosclerosis to try to find genetic markers associated with increased risk. Already, three genetic disorders have been linked to coronary artery disease.

(Despite its name, it does not mean the heart has stopped working.) The two conditions can be related. Some people who survive a heart attack go on to develop heart failure, for instance. Others may develop heart failure without ever having a heart attack. The most common cause of heart failure is multiple heart attacks.

High blood pressure and heart-valve defects can also lead to heart failure. Alcoholism and drug abuse are other causes.

Because the two sides of the heart perform different functions, doctors can often tell which side is failing simply by the symptoms a patient is experiencing. The left side pumps blood that has just been supplied with oxygen from the lungs out into the arteries. If that side isn't performing adequately, blood and fluid can accumulate in the lungs, causing shortness of breath and persistent coughing. The right chambers of the heart receive blood from the body's tissues. If this side is in trouble, fluid and pressure build up in the veins that return blood to the heart. The pressure can cause pain in the liver and swelling in the legs, called edema. This condition is called congestive heart failure.

Other forms of heart trouble

Coronary artery disease is by far the leading form of heart disease, but there are many other types of cardiovascular problems. Here are four of the most common.

HOT TOPIC

Poor Sleepers Beware

Are you a ferocious snorer? Do you wake up feeling exhausted? You may be suffering from sleep apnea—which could be bad news for your heart. In this condition, breathing stops repeatedly for brief periods during the night. People usually wake up during these lapses, although they may not remember doing so. Scientists have found that sleep apnea is associated with increased risk for a variety of cardiovascular diseases, including ischemia (lack of blood and oxygen to the heart) and heartbeat irregularities.

According to a University of Wisconsin study published in *The New England Journal of Medicine* in 2000, people with sleep apnea are much more likely than those who sleep soundly to suffer high blood pressure. It's now thought that nearly 50 percent of sleep apnea patients have hypertension. Those with the most severe sleep apnea seem to have the highest blood pressure—and often the hardest time controlling it. Snoring alone doesn't seem to pose a problem. But if snoring occurs along with sleep apnea—or obesity—the risk of high blood pressure climbs.

Why sleep disorders are linked to heart disease is still something of a mystery. But treating sleep apnea by opening up the airways (usually by wearing a special mask that delivers pressurized air, or through surgery) can bring blood pressure down. If you often wake during the night and feel sleepy during the day, mention your symptoms to your doctor.

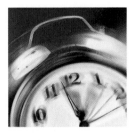

Congenital heart disease. Six to eight babies out of every 1,000 are born with some kind of heart or circulatory defect. Often the cause is unknown, although infections during pregnancy or a mother's use of alcohol, cocaine, or other drugs can damage the heart. Congenital defects are more common in children of mothers with congenital heart problems. Problems can include malformed heart valves, abnormalities that impede the flow of blood through vessels, and defects in the structure of the heart. Congenital heart defects can be diagnosed in utero as early as the sixteenth week of life. Once a baby is born, surgeons are often able to correct the defect.

Cardiomyopathy. Poor nutrition, inflammation caused by viral infections, and complications during pregnancy can cause damage to heart muscle, called cardiomyopathy. This in turn can reduce the heart's pumping efficiency. In 80 percent of cases, physicians are unable to identify a cause. When the cause is unknown, researchers call the condition idiopathic cardiomyopathy. Unlike most other forms of heart disease, this type can affect young people. It is one of the leading causes of sudden cardiac arrest.

Heartbeat irregularities. Almost everyone's heart skips a beat now and then or produces a double beat in the place of a single beat. Most of the time these minor irregularities, called arrhythmias, don't signal trouble. But certain types of arrhythmias caused by coronary artery disease can pose a serious threat. In ventricular fibrillation, for instance, the ventricles (lower chambers of the heart) rapidly contract in an uncoordinated way, causing the heart to stop pumping. Arrhythmias are the leading cause of sudden cardiac death among Americans, accounting for an estimated 400,000 deaths a year. Medications or pacemakers can control many forms of arrhythmias.

Diseases of the heart valves. Four valves control the flow of blood into and out of the heart. Blood entering the heart flows through the tricuspid valve into the right ventricle and, from there, through the pulmonary valve to the lungs, where it picks up oxygen. Returning from the lungs, newly oxygenated blood enters the left atrium and passes through the mitral valve to the left ventricle. It's then pumped through the aortic valve and out into the body. Congenital defects, infections, or the buildup of calcium can interfere with the function of heart valves, making the heart less efficient. Most valve problems can be treated with drugs or repaired with surgery, including the insertion of mechanical valves.

FAST FACT

In 50 percent of men and 63 percent of women who died suddenly of coronary artery disease, there were no previous symptoms of the disease.

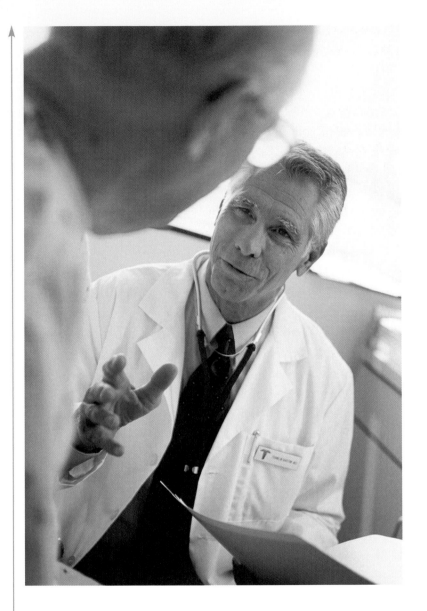

Assessing Your Heart's Condition

The answers to a few simple questions and results of tests done right in your doctor's examining room can provide a surprisingly detailed picture of the state of your heart and your overall health. During the medical interview, your doctor or cardiologist will talk with you about how you're feeling, your family history, and any risk factors you may have. He or she will also want to know what kinds of symptoms you're having. It's essential to answer the questions as completely and honestly as you can and to mention any concerns you have. After all, a symptom you've been experiencing may provide your doctor with a vital clue. That's why it's a good idea to make a list of the things you want to cover and bring it with you, so you don't forget something important.

The physical exam

The goal of a physical exam is to learn as much about what's going on inside the body as possible from the outside. Just looking at skin color, for instance, can tell a doctor whether the heart is delivering enough oxygen to the tissues in the body. Listening through a stethoscope can indicate how the four chambers of the heart are working together. During a physical exam, your doctor will check the health of your heart and blood vessels using five standard tests.

1. Blood pressure. This familiar test uses a cuff wrapped around your upper arm and inflated to create pressure. The cuff is attached to a thermometerlike gauge filled with mercury. By listening to your pulse when the cuff is inflated and then as it is deflated, your physician notes when he can no longer hear the heartbeat and then when it becomes audible again. The mercury level indicates pressure when your heart beats and when it rests.

2. Heart rate and rhythm. By feeling your pulse with his or her fingertips, your doctor can spot signs of an irregular heart rhythm. He or she can also determine your resting heart rate, or the number of times your heart beats each minute.

3. Venous pulses. A doctor can actually see your pulse by looking at a vein on your neck called the jugular. By observing how this vein expands as your heart beats, your doctor can estimate the pressure on the right side of your heart and spot signs that there may be extra fluid in your cardiovascular system.

4. Edema. Excess fluid may accumulate in your legs if your heart isn't pumping effectively. This condition, called edema, can cause visible swelling around your ankles,

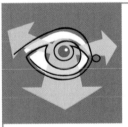

LOOKING AHEAD
Before you have angioplasty

A new test to measure the pressure of blood flow through clogged arteries could help doctors identify patients who would benefit most from treatment. The experimental technique uses a catheter to measure blood flow at the same time an angiogram (see page 54) is performed. Studies have shown that if blood flow is only minimally reduced—even in patients with atherosclerosis—opening up the artery with balloon angioplasty offers no benefit. If blood flow is moderately reduced, however—even if the blockage itself doesn't appear to be substantial—angioplasty can be lifesaving.

TERMS TO KNOW

ANGINA Chest pain or pressure caused by blockage of the arteries that supply blood to the heart

ANGIOGRAM An X-ray test that uses dye injected into blood vessels to create a detailed image of the coronary arteries

ARRHYTHMIA Abnormal heart rhythm

CARDIAC ENZYMES Substances normally found in the heart that can provide a signal when heart muscle is damaged

CARDIOMYOPATHY Any structural or functional disease of the heart muscle

DEFIBRILLATOR A device that delivers an electrical charge designed to "shock" an arrested heart into beating again

ECHOCARDIOGRAM A noninvasive diagnostic test that uses ultrasound waves to create a picture of the heart

EDEMA Swelling caused by the accumulation of fluid, which can be a symptom of heart failure

ELECTROCARDIOGRAM A common diagnostic test that uses electrodes to record the heart's electrical activity

HEART FAILURE A condition in which the heart can no longer pump blood adequately

MYOCARDIAL ISCHEMIA A condition caused when too little blood and oxygen reach the heart muscle as a result of blockage to the arteries

PLAQUE A deposit of fat and other substances in the inner lining of an artery wall

RADIOISOTOPE SCANNING A diagnostic test (also called radionuclide scanning) that uses radioactive dye injected into the bloodstream to create a detailed picture of the heart and arteries

SILENT ISCHEMIA A blockage of blood flow that causes no symptoms

shins, thighs, lower back, abdomen, or hands. To test for fluid retention, your doctor presses on the skin to see how far it can be pushed in, creating an indentation.

5. Heartbeat, breathing, and blood flow. Placing a stethoscope on the skin above your heart, your doctor can gauge how well your heart valves are opening and closing. Telltale sounds called murmurs, snaps, knocks, rubs, and clicks also provide information about possible heart defects. By listening through the stethoscope while you breathe in and out, your doctor is alert to sounds that may indicate that extra fluid has accumulated in your lungs. Placing the stethoscope over other parts of your body, he or she can hear the sound of blood flowing in major vessels. A whispering sound, called bruits, is a sign of abnormal turbulence in blood flow.

Diagnostic Tests

When doctors find signs of trouble during a physical exam, they turn to more sophisticated tests to learn the precise cause, including blood tests and procedures used to create images of the heart and blood vessels.

Secrets from the blood

Human blood reveals an astonishing amount of information about the body, from the state of the immune system to the functioning of organs such as the liver and kidneys. As you've already discovered, a simple blood test can reveal your total, HDL, and LDL cholesterol levels—an important gauge of the health of your blood vessels. Blood tests can also uncover other risk factors, such as abnormal homocysteine levels and the presence of enzymes that signal high levels of inflammation.

If your doctor suspects your heart may have suffered damage as a result of artery blockages, blood tests can indicate the extent of injury. Blood levels of certain heart enzymes rise in the hours following damage to heart muscle. Four cardiac enzymes your doctor may test for are creatine kinase, lactate dehydrogenase, troponin-I, and troponin-T.

Electrocardiograms

The most common test used to diagnose heart conditions is the electrocardiogram, sometimes abbreviated as ECG or EKG.

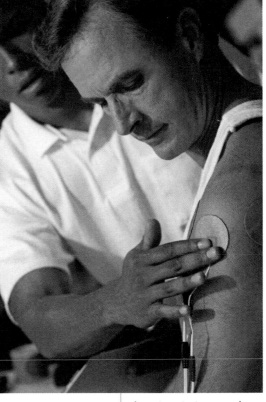

In a stress test, or exercise ECG, a faster heart rate makes it easier to detect ischemia (reduced blood and oxygen supply to the heart) and rhythm abnormalities brought on by exercise.

Both abbreviations refer to the same test. Electrocardiograms can be performed in three basic ways: a resting ECG; an exercise ECG; and an ambulatory, or walking, ECG.

1. Resting ECG. If your doctor suspects heart disease, the first test is likely to be a resting ECG, which creates a graph or tracing of your heart's electrical signals while you remain still.

WHAT TO EXPECT First, electrodes are placed at various locations on your body, usually the ankles, wrists, and chest. They are often covered with a sticky goo that ensures good contact. Wires from the electrodes transmit electrical signals to a small device that creates a tracing of your heart rate and rhythm. The test, which can be done in an examining room, usually takes about 5 minutes.

WHAT THE RESULTS SHOW Electrocardiograms help doctors diagnose irregular heart rhythms, damage from a heart attack, or other heart abnormalities. ECGs can also indicate signs of inadequate blood and oxygen supply to specific regions of heart muscle.

2. Exercise ECG. In some cases, signs and symptoms of heart problems show up during exertion. If the resting ECG fails to show any abnormalities, your doctor may prescribe an exercise ECG, more commonly known as a stress test.

WHAT TO EXPECT Electrodes are attached just as they are for a resting ECG. You'll be asked to walk and then perhaps run on a treadmill to raise your heart rate. The treadmill starts slowly. Gradually the pace and the incline are increased in order to put more demand on your heart. Don't worry: You will be monitored constantly during the test. The moment you feel pain or become tired or too short of breath to continue, the test will be stopped. An exercise ECG, which is usually done in a clinic or hospital, takes about half an hour.

WHAT THE RESULTS SHOW Like a resting ECG, the exercise treadmill test can turn up a variety of abnormalities in heart rhythm. If you experience chest pressure or pain while on the treadmill, the test confirms that you have angina. Your doctor can gauge how severe the angina is, based on how long you remain on the treadmill before the pain occurs.

3. Ambulatory ECG. If you suffer from intermittent heartbeat abnormalities, your doctor may recommend an ambulatory ECG, also sometimes called a Holter monitor. This test records heart activity over a 24-hour period.

WHAT TO EXPECT Electrodes are connected to a recording device about the size of a paperback book, which you'll be asked to wear over 24 hours, even while you sleep. As you go about your everyday business, the device records your heart's electrical patterns. Your doctor may also ask you to keep a diary of what you're doing and any symptoms you experience. Later, technicians will analyze the data, correlating your heartbeat patterns to what you were doing and how you felt.

WHAT THE RESULTS SHOW By providing continuous monitoring of the heart, an ambulatory ECG enables physicians to detect abnormalities that may show up

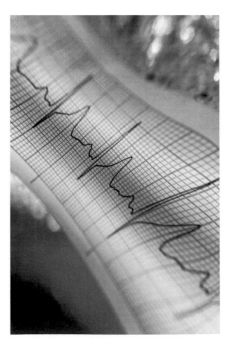

An ECG trace shows the electrical activity of the heart as the upper chamber contracts, then the lower. In between beats, the heart rests.

only once in a while in a 24-hour period. It also allows them to see how specific activities affect your heart, providing important clues about which ones trigger abnormal heart rhythms, for instance.

Electrophysiologic tests

Like an ECG, an electrophysiologic test uses electrodes to measure electrical signals emanating from the heart. Instead of being placed on the skin, however, the electrodes are inserted through veins and sometimes arteries directly into the heart's chambers to record electrical signals from within the heart. Consequently, this is considered a more invasive procedure. Cardiologists sometimes intentionally trigger abnormal heart rhythms in order to gauge whether a particular drug or surgical repair will help stop the disturbance. Electrophysiologic tests are sometimes used when ECG results are inconclusive.

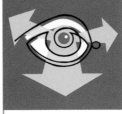

LOOKING AHEAD
The closest look yet inside arteries

A new form of high-resolution magnetic resonance imaging (MRI) recently created the most detailed images ever recorded of the inside of coronary arteries in living patients. The technology can be used to pinpoint potential trouble spots in arteries long before symptoms of atherosclerosis show up, say researchers at Mount Sinai School of Medicine in New York. Experts hope the technique, called "black blood MRI," will allow doctors to identify vulnerable artery plaques before they rupture. They could then more precisely target treatments to prevent heart attacks. Although promising, the test remains experimental.

WHAT TO EXPECT The test is usually performed in a special office or laboratory. The area where the electrode catheters will be inserted (usually the groin) is scrubbed and shaved. Typically, three or four catheters—each one about as big around as a strand of spaghetti—are inserted at the same time. If your doctor uses a small electrical charge to trigger an arrhythmia, you may feel an unusual heartbeat or a fluttering feeling in your heart. When the test begins, the table you are lying on will be horizontal. During the test, it may be tilted to an upright position so that your doctor can assess your heart's response to changes in position. The process can take anywhere from one hour to more than four hours.

WHAT THE RESULTS SHOW Electrophysiologic studies produce a map of the heart's electrical system, showing how nerve impulses are conducted from one part of the heart to another. They help doctors determine where along the conduction system the electrical impulses that produce your heartbeat are going awry and which treatments can be used to fix the problem.

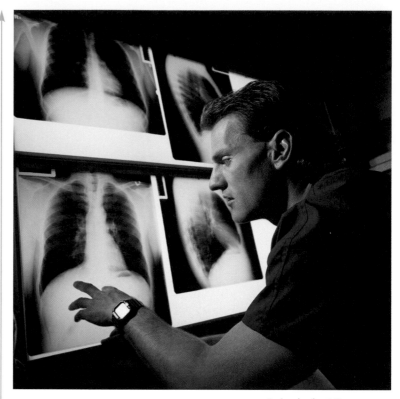

A simple chest X ray can reveal calcium deposits, heart enlargement, and lung changes caused by heart failure.

Imaging techniques

Doctors have at their disposal a variety of tools for creating images of the heart and circulatory system, from simple X rays to highly sophisticated tests that provide three-dimensional and even moving pictures of the heart. The imaging tests your doctor is most likely to recommend include:

1. Chest X ray. A chest X ray, just like the kind used to see the condition of your lungs, can provide important clues to the state of your heart.

WHAT TO EXPECT After removing clothes and jewelry above your waist, you'll stand against a plate that contains X-ray film. X rays will be aimed at your chest. They penetrate different tissues in different ways, creating an image of bone, heart muscle, and the outline of your lungs on X-ray film.

WHAT THE RESULTS SHOW X rays provide a picture of the size and shape of your heart. They can also reveal calcium

TROUBLESHOOTING TIP

Diagnostic tests can be scary. Remember:
■ If you have questions about why a test is being ordered, ask your doctor.
■ If you're worried about what a test will be like, ask for a description of exactly what will be done and how it will feel.
■ If you find yourself very anxious about a test, say so. Your doctor may be able to give you medication to help you calm down.

deposits that may indicate heart disease or injury, as well as provide information about the health of your lungs.

2. Radioisotope scanning. Like X rays, radioisotope scans use very low levels of radiation to create images of the heart. But while an X ray creates a picture by passing radiation through the body from an outside source, a radioisotope scan uses radioactive material injected into the bloodstream. Special cameras detect the material as it passes through the heart and arteries, providing vital information about coronary blood flow.

DIAGNOSING A STROKE

A stroke occurs when blood supply to parts of the brain is interrupted. There are two main types of stroke. In an ischemic stroke, blood flow is blocked as a result of atherosclerosis, sometimes compounded by a blood clot. Hemorrhagic strokes occur when a blood vessel in the brain ruptures. A variety of tests allow doctors to zero in on the area of the brain that was affected and assess the kind of damage that occurred.

■ **Taking pictures.** Several of the same tests that help doctors diagnose heart disease can detect strokes. CT, or computed tomography, scans, for instance, are used to determine the kind of stroke and where it has occurred. MRIs create highly detailed images of the brain, pinpointing the location and size of the affected area. Angiograms very similar to those used to create an image of the coronary arteries can also be used to make detailed maps of blood flow in the brain, showing which areas have been robbed of blood supply.

■ **Tracing electrical activity.** Doctors can also trace the brain's electrical activity with an electroencephalogram, or EEG. Electrodes placed at strategic locations on the scalp detect electrical impulses in various parts of the brain. By recording the intensity, duration, frequency, and location of electrical activity, EEGs help doctors assess the damage.

■ **Listening in.** Tests that measure sound waves also provide important clues. A device that emits ultrasound, for instance, can be used to record the speed of blood cells flowing through the carotid arteries, the two main vessels that supply blood to the brain. In another test, called a carotid phonoangiogram, doctors place a small microphone against the neck to record the sound of blood flowing through these arteries. The microphone is sensitive enough to pick up the difference between normal blood flow and the sound of turbulence that may indicate a blockage.

WHAT TO EXPECT Although the injection of radioactive material sounds a little scary, it's very safe. The amount of radiation is roughly what you receive during a standard chest X ray. The material, called a tracer, is injected into your arm. The test may be performed while you are resting, or you may be asked to exercise on a treadmill or stationary bike before the tracer material is injected. Afterward you'll lie still while a camera takes a series of pictures from different angles, which can last up to 25 minutes. This type of test is more accurate than an exercise ECG and sometimes used when the results of an ECG are inconclusive or when more information is needed. It is also considerably more expensive.

WHAT THE RESULTS SHOW The detailed images of your heart and the blood vessels that supply it can reveal the extent of damage to heart muscles after a heart attack or measure the amount of blood that passes through the heart each time it beats. A form of radioisotope scanning called single photon emission computed tomography (SPECT) can be used to create a three-dimensional functional image of the heart. These scans are extremely accurate in detecting ischemias, or areas of restricted blood flow.

3. Coronary Angiography. Angiography involves the injection of a special dye into the arteries that supply the heart, allowing the heart's activity to be recorded by X-ray cameras. This is the most common test used to diagnose coronary artery disease. Angiography can reveal blockages or narrowed areas that aren't visible on normal X rays.

WHAT TO EXPECT A narrow tube called a catheter is inserted into an artery in the groin. Alternatively it may be inserted at the wrist or elbow. A local anesthetic is used to numb the area. The catheter is fed through the artery until it reaches a coronary artery. Dye is injected, and a series of X rays is taken. The insertion of the

Coronary angiography reveals sections of arteries that have been narrowed by coronary artery disease.

catheter is usually painless. Some patients experience a few palpitations when the tube reaches the heart. The test, which takes about 40 minutes, is usually done as an outpatient procedure. The injection site may be bruised and tender for a few days.

WHAT THE RESULTS SHOW An angiogram of the heart provides a detailed image of the condition of the vessels that supply blood to the heart, including any blockages. Angiography is typically used when doctors believe a patient may benefit from heart surgery or angioplasty, a technique that opens blocked vessels.

4. Echocardiography. Echocardiography offers a noninvasive way to look at your heart. Instead of X rays and dyes, it uses echoes. Sound waves, called ultrasound, are directed at the heart via a microphonelike device called a transducer. By detecting the echoes that bounce back from the heart, echocardiography traces a picture of your heart while it is beating.

WHAT TO EXPECT An echocardiogram can be done in a cardiologist's office or at a hospital. The doctor or technician will apply gel or oil to your chest to improve the transmission of ultrasound waves. The test is usually painless, although sometimes the transducer must be held very firmly against the skin, which can feel a bit uncomfortable. Echocardiography typically takes about 15 minutes to an hour.

WHAT THE RESULTS SHOW The images produced by an echocardiogram can reveal damage to the heart muscle, valve problems, abnormal blood flow, and other conditions.

Advanced imaging techniques

Several tests can create even more detailed images of the heart, including three-dimensional pictures. These include computed tomography (CT), magnetic resonance imaging (MRI), and positron emission tomography (PET). New advances are making

Key Finding

Research shows that a new form of high-resolution magnetic resonance imaging (MRI) can detect most diseased coronary arteries, possibly sparing patients from undergoing an angiogram, a more invasive test. MRI has been used to examine very large blood vessels for years. But only recently has it been adapted to produce images of the relatively small coronary arteries. According to a study published in the December 2001 issue of *The New England Journal of Medicine,* the so-called ultrafast MRI detected every diseased coronary artery in 75 percent of patients studied. It ruled out coronary artery disease accurately between 81 percent and 100 percent of the time. An added bonus: MRI costs about $1,000, compared with about $5,000 for an angiogram.

them more accurate than ever. CT scans use X rays, but instead of taking a single picture, the X-ray machine is rotated rapidly around the body so that images are captured from all angles. This allows doctors to view internal organs in cross section. An even newer test called cine-computed tomography creates a three-dimensional moving image of the heart. MRIs record small energy signals emitted by the atoms that make up cells in different body tissues. PET scans, the newest diagnostic tool, and one that is currently used mostly for research purposes, detect emissions from subatomic particles. They can determine how well portions of the heart muscle are functioning after a heart attack, helping doctors decide whether or not to repair a blockage of an artery supplying blood to that area.

WHAT TO EXPECT You'll lie flat on a movable table. In a CT scan, the table is passed slowly through a giant ring that scans your body from all angles. In an MRI scan, the table is moved through a stationary chamber. You'll be required to lie very still while inside the magnetic chamber. The operation of the magnet is very noisy. The procedure, which is painless, can take half an hour or more. In a PET scan, a small amount of radioactive material is injected into the blood before the scan, which takes about an hour.

WHAT THE RESULTS SHOW High-tech scans can be used to evaluate ischemia and look at diseases of the heart valves.

An ounce of prevention

The diagnostic tests now available provide an astonishingly clear portrait of the state of the heart and circulatory system, helping doctors pinpoint the source of trouble so they can treat it more effectively. That's excellent news, of course. But researchers also hope that they can encourage people to prevent cardiovascular problems from developing in the first place. One of the best ways to do that is to stop smoking. Turn the page to learn more.

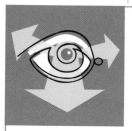

LOOKING AHEAD
Early warning sign of heart attack

Researchers may soon be able to identify plaques on arteries that are vulnerable to rupturing and blocking blood flow, possibly triggering a heart attack. In 2001, researchers at Germany's Bonn University injected into the bloodstream magnetic molecules that bind to fibrin, a substance that forms in plaques. MRI scans were then used to spot where the molecules had accumulated. The technique could one day help doctors determine the degree of danger and guide them in deciding how to treat patients with vulnerable plaques.

REAL PEOPLE, REAL WISDOM

A Doctor's Story

The signs of trouble were there, Stephen Weiss, M.D., realizes, if only he'd been paying enough attention to notice them. "I realize now that for almost two years I'd been experiencing what doctors call exertional angina—chest pain that comes on during physical

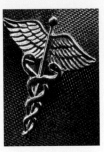

exertion," says Dr. Weiss, 46, a general practitioner in northern California. "My chest would feel tight, and I'd be short of breath after climbing hills on my bicycle. But frankly, I figured I was just getting older."

Then after a bout of the flu, Dr. Weiss noticed he was having much more than the usual trouble getting back in shape. Simply walking to another department during work, he experienced pain and tightness in his chest.

It wasn't until a few days later, at home, that he realized something was seriously wrong. "I'd gone out to get a package, and by the time I got back inside I was so weak I had to lie down on the floor." His wife insisted he go to the emergency room, where he was examined by a cardiologist. "At first glance everything looked normal. My blood pressure. My pulse rate. The chest X ray. My cardiac C-reactive enzymes. My cholesterol levels."

The cardiologist conducted a stress test, or treadmill electrocardiogram. Three months earlier, Dr. Weiss had completed a three-hour bike ride with no trouble. Now he could barely last for 10 minutes on the treadmill. The cardiologist ordered an angiogram, a test that

uses injected dye to create a detailed image of the arteries that supply the heart. When Dr. Weiss saw the results, he knew he was lucky to be alive. One of his coronary arteries was almost 99 percent blocked. At any time, a blood clot could have closed it off completely, triggering a heart attack.

Finally the cardiologist performed an angioplasty, which uses a small inflated balloon to widen the blocked vessel. Then a metal device called a stent was inserted to help prevent the artery from closing up again.

Six months later, Dr. Weiss is working full-time again and beginning to return to his normal activity level. But things aren't the same. For starters, he and his family have dramatically changed the way they eat, adopting a low-fat regimen with much more fruit, vegetables, and whole-grain foods. The goal: to reverse some of the damage of coronary artery disease by following a strict diet and getting back to exercise. He's also become serious about controlling stress by finding time for himself and using relaxation techniques like meditation on a regular basis.

"It's been scary," he admits. "But it's also made me a different and, I hope, a better doctor. I find myself spending a little more time with my patients, listening more closely to what they're telling me. I missed the first signs that something was wrong with me. I don't want to miss them in my patients."

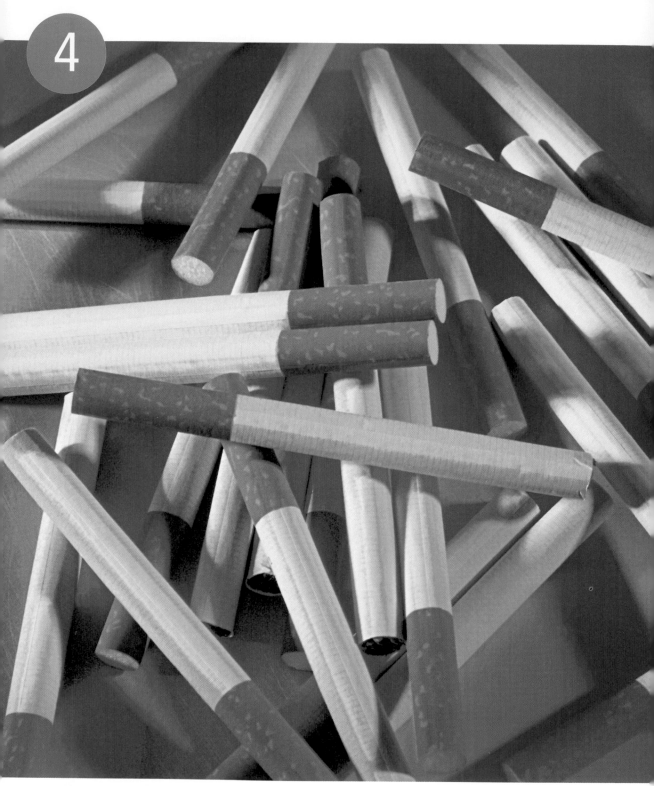

4

Kicking the Habit

Smoking is bad for your body, and your heart is no exception. The nasty habit can raise your blood pressure, narrow your blood vessels, wreak havoc on your ratio of "good" cholesterol to "bad" cholesterol, and put you at higher risk of blood clots that cause heart attacks and strokes, to name just some of the dangers. The good news: Even if you've been a long-term smoker, you can substantially cut your risk of premature death by quitting today.

Chances are you'd like to stop smoking. In fact, at any given moment, four out of five smokers say they want to do just that. But we know that stamping out a tobacco addiction is anything but easy. On the other hand, as more than a million smokers prove every year, it can be done.

If you've tried and failed to quit, take heart: Most people attempt to give up smoking two or three times before they succeed for good. Those early efforts aren't failures; they're more like dress rehearsals—a chance to figure out which strategies work for you. And quitting today is easier than ever before thanks to a variety of smoking-cessation aids, from nicotine patches and gum to medication that takes the edge off of cravings.

The payoffs of quitting are enormous. You'll start enjoying some of them right away. Food will taste better. Your mouth will feel fresher. You'll begin to have more energy. More important, after one year of being smoke-free, your excess risk of heart disease will fall by half. Three to four years after you quit, you'll be at no greater risk than someone who has never smoked.

> "Three to four years after you quit, you'll be at no greater risk of heart disease than someone who has never smoked."

Hard Habit to Break

Why are cigarettes so difficult to jettison? First, nicotine is physically addictive. For some people it can be as addictive as heroine or cocaine, according to the U.S. Public Health Service. When smokers try to quit, they may feel irritable, light-headed, and anxious. Many have trouble concentrating for the first week or two.

Second, smoking becomes tied to one's daily routines, creating a psychological dependence. Lighting up may be part of the morning ritual, for instance. Many smokers associate smoking with meals and find themselves craving a cigarette after lunch or dinner. These obstacles can also be overcome. By changing your routines and avoiding situations you associate with smoking, you can steer clear of psychological triggers.

A weighty matter

One reason some people hesitate to quit is a fear of weight gain. Not everyone who gives up smoking will pay for it at the scale. But on average, smokers who quit put on between 7 and 14 pounds during the first six months after stopping. Scientists don't fully understand why. One explanation may simply be that food tastes better after you get rid of the taste of smoke in your mouth, so your appetite increases. Another may be that smoking revs up your metabolism, which causes the body to burn extra calories. When you quit, your metabolism cranks down just a bit.

All else being equal, scientists estimate that the average person burns about 200 more calories a day when smoking than when not. How can you make up the difference? One brisk 30-minute walk will do the trick. Or pass up a single high-calorie snack, like a candy bar. Finally, remember that it's far better to carry a few extra pounds than to poison your body with tobacco and suffer all the attendant harms.

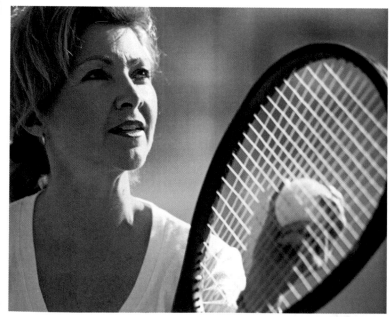

Exercise can offset any weight gain associated with kicking the habit. And studies show it can boost your chances of success.

Twelve reasons to quit

Not sure you're ready to throw those cigarettes away? The first step in making any lasting change is convincing yourself that the benefits are worth the effort. With smoking, that shouldn't be difficult. Consider these incentives.

1. You'll live longer. Men who quit before the age of 39 add an average five years to their lives. Women gain an additional three years. Even smokers who wait until their 60s to quit live an extra year longer.

2. You'll have more energy and stamina to do the things you enjoy.

3. You'll look better. Smoking yellows the teeth and causes premature wrinkling and drying of the skin.

4. Smoking is the leading cause of lung cancer, emphysema, and bronchitis.

5. When you light up, you expose the people you love to the hazards of secondhand smoke. According to one estimate, 35,000 to 40,000 cases of heart disease in nonsmokers are caused by secondhand smoke each year.

6. Smoking reduces the proportion of LDL ("bad cholesterol") to HDL ("good cholesterol").

7. Smoking generates free radicals, unstable molecules that oxidize deposits of cholesterol on the lining of blood vessel walls, making them more likely to rupture and cause heart attacks.

8. Nicotine raises blood pressure by 15 to 25 points after you inhale a cigarette.

9. Smoking raises the risk of blood clots that cause heart attacks.

10. Smoking temporarily narrows the blood vessels, increasing the likelihood that coronary arteries already constricted by

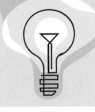

ASK THE EXPERT

Is smoking a cigar safer than smoking cigarettes?

Carlos Iribarren, M.D., MPH, Ph.D., assistant adjunct professor, Department of Epidemiology and Biostatistics, University of California San Francisco School of Medicine:

"This question is a little like asking if jumping out of a fourth-story window is safer than jumping out of an eighth-story window. Both can kill you.

Some people think smoking cigars is safer than cigarettes because most cigar smokers don't inhale. But surveys show that 10 percent of cigar puffers do inhale. Even those who don't, breathe in plenty of secondhand smoke. Plus they swallow a witches' brew of toxic substances from cigar smoke, which includes more nicotine, benzene, lead-nitrogen oxides, and other harmful chemicals than cigarette smoke contains.

People who smoke cigars don't tend to do so as often as cigarette smokers. But in a study we conducted at the University of California, we found a higher risk of heart disease, chronic pulmonary disease, and cancers of the mouth, esophagus, and lungs among men who regularly puffed cigars than those who didn't. Drinking alcohol seemed to increase the danger."

atherosclerosis will become so obstructed that angina or a heart attack results.

11. In men smoking can lead to impotence.

12. If you smoke, your children are much more likely to take up the cigarette habit.

A Quitter's Game Plan

When you decide you're ready to kick the habit, make an appointment with your doctor to discuss your decision to quit. Why? First, studies have shown that person-to-person tobacco dependence counseling, either one-on-one or through a group, boosts your chances of success. Your doctor can help you tailor a program to fit your needs. Second, he or she can help you decide whether to use a medication designed to smooth the way and write a prescription if one is necessary.

Five such drugs have been approved by the U.S. Food and Drug Administration. Some people use just one; others combine two. Four of the drugs are alternative nicotine-delivery systems that send a controlled amount of nicotine to your brain to satisfy your craving for the substance without the drawbacks of tobacco. They include a nasal spray, an inhaler, a gum, and a patch. An analysis conducted in 2000 found that people on nicotine-replacement therapy increased their odds of quitting by 70 percent.

SMOKING-CESSATION AIDS

These drugs can significantly boost your chances of quitting. All of them have potential (usually mild) side effects. Talk to your doctor about which ones might be right for you.

MEDICATION	SIDE EFFECTS	DURATION	AVAILABILITY	COST PER DAY
Sustained-release bupropion (Zyban)	Insomnia, dry mouth	7 to 12 weeks; maintenance, up to 6 months	Prescription only	$3.33
Nicotine gum	Mouth soreness, dyspepsia	Up to 12 weeks	Over-the-counter	$6.25 for 10 2-mg pieces
Nicotine inhaler	Mouth and throat irritation	Up to 6 months	Prescription only	$5.40 for 12 doses
Nicotine nasal spray	Nasal irritation	3 to 6 months	Prescription only	$5.40 for 12 doses
Nicotine patch	Local skin reaction	8 weeks	Prescription and over-the-counter	$3.75

Can Hypnosis or Acupuncture Help?

Some people swear by these approaches, claiming they've helped them to stop smoking, even after just one session. Others say they're bogus. What's the real truth?

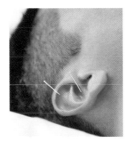

Hypnotic suggestion has been used for decades to help smokers give up cigarettes. But even the experts can't agree on whether it works.

On the positive side, researchers at Ohio State University interviewed 452 people who had participated in a group-hypnotherapy smoking-cessation program sponsored by the American Lung Association of Ohio. Five to 15 months after attending the single-day program, 22 percent of the participants said they had not smoked in the preceding month. Hypnosis, the researchers concluded, offers a reasonable alternative to other smoking-cessation methods.

But not everyone is convinced. When researchers from the University of Leicester, in England, analyzed nine studies that used hypnosis to enable smokers to quit, they found no evidence that this method helped.

The verdict on acupuncture is just as mixed. The ancient healing practice involves the insertion of small needles just below the surface of the skin at specific sites on the body, such as the earlobes, chest, or arms.

Some studies have shown real benefit. At the University of Oslo, in Norway, researchers divided 46 men and 39 women randomly into two groups. One group received acupuncture at locations on their bodies traditionally identified as antismoking points. The other received a placebo treatment: needles inserted at random locations not associated with addiction. Volunteers in both groups reduced the number of cigarettes smoked each day. But 31 percent of the smokers receiving genuine acupuncture managed to quit successfully during the course of the study. Not one of those in the fake acupuncture group was able to quit for good.

A 1998 British study turned up similar positive results. In an experiment involving 78 smokers, 12.5 percent of those in the acupuncture group had successfully quit after six months compared with none in the control group.

But not all the reports are encouraging. In 2001, researchers in Germany reviewed 39 studies of the benefits of acupuncture. They found no convincing evidence that genuine acupuncture was any better than sham acupuncture in smoking cessation.

What's the bottom line? If you're determined to give acupuncture or hypnosis a try, look for a practitioner associated with a local hospital or medical center. That way you're more likely to find someone with bona fide credentials. If you haven't quit smoking within a month, it's time to choose another approach.

CALIFORNIA STRIKES GOLD

In 1989 the California government created the California Tobacco Control Program to reduce smoking rates. One of its strategies was to "denormalize" tobacco by countering the advertising images of smoking as glamorous and sexy with images of the real costs of smoking. In one famous ad the Marlboro man is seen puffing on a drooping cigarette—a reference to the fact that smoking can cause impotence in men. In another a group of tobacco-company executives meet in a smoke-filled room, plotting ways to find new customers to replace the old ones—who died from smoking.

The campaign worked. According to a 2001 report, one million fewer Californians smoke as a result of the state's efforts. Per capita cigarette consumption has been cut in half. Lives are being saved every day. But experts from the California Department of Health Services warn that the tobacco industry is "still aggressively marketing their products to teenagers, ethnic minority groups, and young adults."

You can use the same technique California employed to help yourself quit: Create a mental image of smoking as dirty, smelly, and unpleasant to people around you. If that's not enough, mentally associate cigarettes with those executives in that smoke-filled room who have used every trick in the book to hook you on this addictive and potentially lethal product. Don't let them keep you enslaved to nicotine.

View smoking as a dirty, dangerous habit, and you'll be less tempted to light up.

The fifth smoking-cessation aid is a prescription medication called Zyban (bupropion). Scientists aren't sure why it quells the craving, but several studies have shown that it can boost many people's chances of quitting. In a 2001 study from the Mayo Clinic's Nicotine Dependence Center, a group of 784 smokers were given sustained-release Zyban along with counseling. After seven weeks, 461 had beaten their addiction. Those people were then divided into two groups—one received Zyban for 45 weeks, the others a placebo. A year after the study began, 55 percent of the people in the first group were still smoke-free compared with only 42 percent of those in the second. Note that Zyban used in conjunction with a nicotine patch can raise blood pressure. Make sure to have your pressure checked frequently if you're using both.

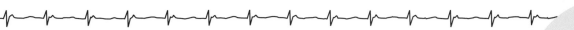

Countdown to quitting

Once you've talked to your doctor, it's time to gear up for the big day when you'll give tobacco the boot. Most experts recommend spending a week or so getting ready. (If you're a very heavy smoker, however, you may want to wean yourself down to a pack a day gradually before you try to quit. One way to do this is by smoking one less cigarette each day.) During this preparation period, you solidify your resolve and gain skills that will help you stop for good.

Quit day minus five

● Fill out the Commit to Quit form on page 66. Post it on your refrigerator or in your office or both.

● Tell friends and family that you've decided to quit.

● To celebrate your decision, smoke one less cigarette today than you did yesterday.

● If you've decided to use Zyban, begin taking the medication as directed by your doctor.

● Make an appointment with your dentist to have your teeth cleaned on quit day minus one.

Quit day minus four

● Start keeping a daily log of when and why you smoke. To help yourself remember, fold the sheet of paper you use for the log around your pack of cigarettes and secure it with a rubber band so that you have to unfold the paper to get a cigarette. Be sure to record things that trigger smoking, such as meals, certain surroundings, or stressful situations.

● Make a list of habits or routines you may want to change to make quitting easier. For example, if you usually have a cigarette with your morning coffee, consider drinking your coffee on the go instead or switching to tea.

TROUBLESHOOTING TIP

To boost your chances of success, pick a good time to quit. Holidays, difficult periods at work, and other stressful circumstances can weaken your resolve. Choose a time when you can really focus on your goal.

COMMIT TO QUIT

Use this form to put your commitment to quitting—and your strategies to make it happen—in writing. Post it where you'll see it often.

I commit to quit on _____ (date).

My top five strategies for quitting (including any medications you intend to use to help you quit) are:

❧ _____

❧ _____

❧ _____

❧ _____

❧ _____

I anticipate the most difficult times will be:

❧ _____

❧ _____

❧ _____

❧ _____

❧ _____

Three people I can turn to for support are:

❧ _____

❧ _____

❧ _____

My three most important reasons for quitting are:

❧ _____

❧ _____

❧ _____

Signed:

_____

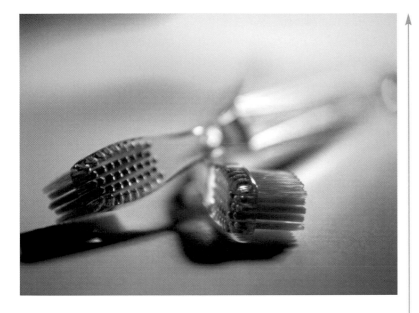

- Plan alternative ways to relax, including simple deep-breathing exercises or even a humorous website you can log onto any time.
- Think of items you can hold in your hand instead of a cigarette, like a pencil, a chopstick, or a squeezable stress-relief ball.
- Smoke one less cigarette than you did yesterday.
- Brush your teeth four times today and appreciate how clean and fresh your mouth tastes afterward.

Quit day minus three

- Write down the names of two or three people you can call on when you need moral support—and let them know they're on your list.
- Think of something you can buy yourself as a reward with the money you save on cigarettes over the next two weeks.
- Continue brushing your teeth four times a day.
- Smoke one less cigarette today than you did yesterday.

Quit day minus two

- Buy nicotine gum or whichever smoking-cessation aid you've decided to use, if you've decided to use one.
- Wash your clothes to get rid of that nasty cigarette odor.
- Brush your teeth four times a day.
- Smoke one less cigarette today than you did yesterday.

TROUBLESHOOTING TIP

The immediate need for a cigarette can seem overpowering, but cravings typically persist only about five minutes. The trick is to outlast them. When a craving hits, make a phone call—even if it's just to make an appointment or check your bank balance. Chances are the urge will subside by the time you hang up.

Quit day minus one

- At the end of the day, throw away all cigarettes and matches and put everything that reminds you of smoking—ashtrays and lighters—out of sight. Remove the lighter from your car.
- Remind friends, family, and coworkers that tomorrow is the day you plan to quit.
- Stock up on hard candies, gum, pumpkin seeds, cinnamon sticks, or whatever else might distract you from smoking.
- Go to your dentist and have your teeth cleaned. Keep them clean by brushing them several times during the day.
- Smoke one less cigarette today than you did yesterday.

Quit day

- Stay busy. Be sure to plan enough activities today to keep yourself plenty distracted.
- Alter your routine to avoid situations in which you would normally smoke. If you usually smoked during your lunch hour, take a brisk walk instead. If possible, avoid the person with whom you used to share your cigarette break.
- Remind yourself of your list of things to do when the craving strikes and be prepared to do them.
- Avoid alcohol if it makes you want to smoke.
- Do something nice for yourself to celebrate your first smoke-free day.
- If you don't manage to get through the whole day without a cigarette, don't despair. Quitting is an ongoing project, not a onetime event.

Key Finding

A program of vigorous exercise can help women both quit smoking and keep weight off, a 1999 study at Brown University School of Medicine found. Researchers divided 281 sedentary smokers into two groups. One group enrolled in a smoking-cessation program. The other combined the same program with three supervised exercise programs a week. Those in the exercise group were more than twice as likely to be smoke-free at the end of 12 months. They had also gained less weight than the non-exercisers.

Taming Temptation

You'll need plenty of willpower—and a little ingenuity—to resist the desire to light up. Think of it as a creative challenge. To get you started, here are 11 tried-and-true temptation fighters.

1. Go somewhere else. Avoid places that serve as triggers for smoking. When the urge to smoke strikes, escape to a smoke-free environment like a library, church, museum, or store. Head to the

REAL PEOPLE, REAL WISDOM

The Power of Persistence

"It's been a rocky road," says Mark Licher, 53, a kitchen designer in Cedar Rapids, Iowa. Licher first decided to kick the habit three years ago, after smoking since the age of 16. "I'd remarried not long before, and my wife had taken up cigarettes again, mostly because I was smoking. I didn't want either of us to smoke. So I decided it was time to quit."

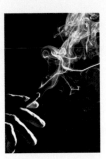

The first time around, using the nicotine patch, Licher made it for six months. Then, like many would-be quitters, the stresses and strains of everyday life derailed him. "My kids, who are mostly grown up now, were having one problem after another. They were in and out of the house. On one particularly bad day I reached for a cigarette. I wasn't smoking as consistently as I had before or as much. But I was smoking again."

A few months later, Licher decided to try once more, this time with the help of acupuncture. It wasn't long before he hit another rough patch with the kids, and he found himself lighting up. After that, he underwent hypnosis and used the non-nicotine drug bupropion, without much success.

"At least I was trying. I was committed. I hadn't given up," says Licher. The kids are out of the house once again, and life has settled down—and it's been just about six months since he's smoked a cigarette.

"I'm following all the advice. I gave up coffee because I've always associated that with cigarettes. I've changed the route I take to work for the same reason. I'm exercising on the treadmill at home because I know that helps. The best thing is that I'm feeling better. Quitting has made a big difference in my physical well-being, in the way I feel when I breathe, and in the energy I have. And believe me, that's something I don't want to give up now just for a puff on a cigarette."

movies for the ultimate distraction, and you'll be assured about two hours without a cigarette.

2. Chomp on carrots or celery sticks. Crunching on either not only helps satisfy the oral craving but also gives you something to do with your hands.

3. Chew gum. Many smokers find chewing gum satisfies the urge to put a cigarette between their lips. If you're worried about weight gain, choose a sugar-free gum or hard candy.

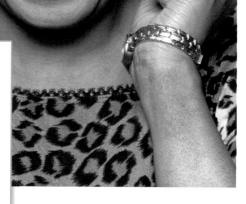

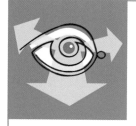

LOOKING AHEAD

A shot to help you quit?

Researchers at the National Institute on Drug Abuse in Bethesda are exploring the possibility of a vaccine to help smokers free themselves from nicotine addiction. Although no such vaccine has yet been tested in smokers, researchers say that immunizations could be used to block or reduce the intake of nicotine into the brain, thus reducing its addictive power. An antismoking vaccine could help prevent adolescent puffers from becoming confirmed smokers. It could also help keep former smokers from relapsing.

4. Get up and get moving. Take a walk around the block, do 20 jumping jacks, hop on your bike or exercise cycle and work up a sweat. Exercise can take the edge off nicotine cravings and also help keep off unwanted pounds. Joining a gym will give you a nonsmoking place to go and something new to focus on.

5. Eat several small meals instead of one big one. Eating mutes the oral craving for cigarettes. If you're eating or drinking, you have less urge to smoke. Also, having smaller meals and eating more frequently keeps your blood sugar levels steady so you don't overeat, which can help you avoid gaining weight.

6. **Call a friend.** Don't be embarrassed to say, "Help! I'm faltering." Good friends or loved ones will do all they can to encourage or distract you.

7. **Practice breathing exercises.** Find a quiet spot to sit, close your eyes, and relax by inhaling and exhaling slowly a dozen times. Breathe from your abdomen, not your chest. Doing this can help short-circuit the urge to light up.

8. **Take a warm shower or bath.** This is an excellent way to release tension and quell the craving for cigarettes. Smoking and water don't mix.

9. **Wash the dishes.** Likewise, it's almost impossible to smoke and have your hands plunged in soapy water. And there's an added benefit: a clean kitchen!

10. **Hold a pencil or even a candy cigarette.** Having something in your hand will make you less likely to reach for a cigarette.

11. **Brush your teeth.** The fresh clean taste in your mouth may well discourage you from polluting it with cigarette smoke.

If at first you don't succeed...

You're not alone. Most long-term smokers try to quit several times before they succeed. Remember that every attempt you make brings you one step closer to your goal. If you do have a lapse, remind yourself that giving in to the urge to smoke a cigarette once or even twice doesn't mean you've failed completely. Too often, people who are trying to make any kind of lasting change in their lives have an all-or-nothing attitude. If they can't kick the habit once and for all, they consider themselves defeated. That kind of thinking turns a momentary slip into a full-scale collapse.

If you falter along the way, don't panic. Instead:

- Remember your three top reasons for wanting to quit.
- Think about what made you smoke that cigarette.
- Write down at least two strategies that will help you over come this obstacle next time you encounter it (look back at your "Commit to Quit" form for ideas).
- Set a new quit date within the coming week.
- Tell at least two friends or family members about your resolution to try again.

The quicker you get back in the game, the better your chances of quitting for good—and the sooner you'll begin to enjoy the benefits of a smoke-free life.

Don't Go It Alone

All kinds of resources out there are devoted to helping you quit smoking. For more information, check out:

✔ **American Cancer Society**
1-800-ACS-2345
www.acs.org

✔ **American Heart Association**
1-800-AHA-USA1
www.amheart.org

✔ **American Lung Association**
1-800-586-4872
www.lungusa.org

✔ **Cessation programs** offered by your local hospital or medical clinic, the local health department, or your health insurance plan

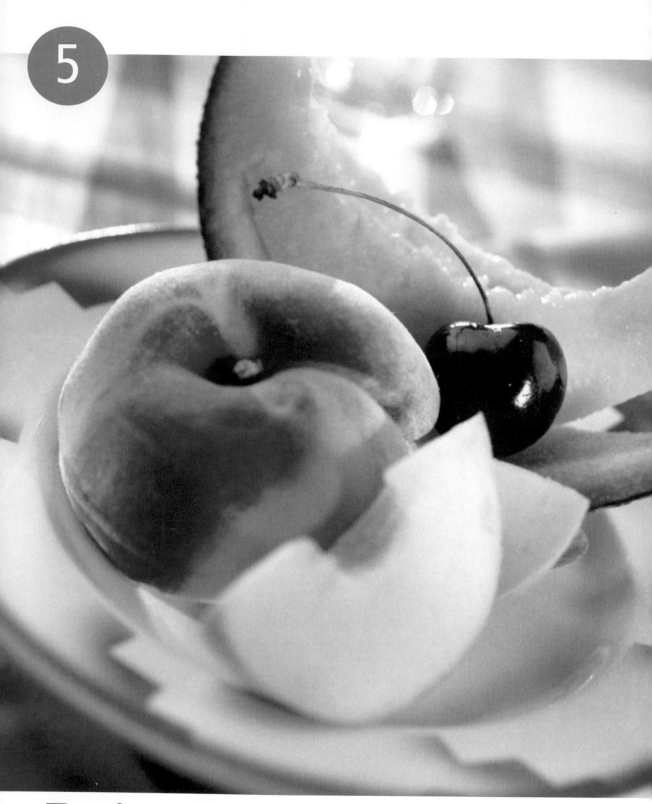

5

Eating Heart Smart

Food lovers, rejoice! The old advice for eating heart smart has been replaced by a new message: Not all fat is bad for your heart. In fact, some of it, like that contained in olive or peanut oil, is actually good for you. Today many foods once banished from a healthy diet, such as nuts and avocados, have been welcomed back onto the menu. The emphasis has shifted from what you shouldn't eat to what you can and should enjoy—delicious foods that help protect your heart.

And what a feast it is. Whole-grain cereals, oatmeal, ripe berries, hearty dark breads, salmon, tuna, lean meats, luscious tomatoes, savory onions, bright orange squash, fresh leafy greens, even a glass of your favorite wine—they're all part of a diet that's as great tasting as it is good for your heart. So enjoy! Because in truth, the heart healthy diet is not about deprivation—it's about eating well.

The Secrets of a Healthy Diet

If, like many Americans, you greet the latest dietary advice with, well, a grain of salt, it's no wonder. Nutrition recommendations have made some confusing flip-flops in recent years. One day the experts tell us to eat a low-fat, high-carbohydrate diet; the next, it seems, they warn that too many carbohydrates may be dangerous. For years we were told that margarine is a better choice than butter. Then along comes news that even margarine contains artery-clogging fats. Meanwhile, dozens of new titles crowd bookstore shelves every year, each one purporting to reveal, at long last, the secret of a healthy diet.

The real secret is this: The basics of a heart healthy diet aren't complicated. And despite the highly publicized reversals, they are rock solid. They boil down to just five pieces of advice:

1. Replace saturated fat with unsaturated fat whenever you can.
2. Go easy on foods high in cholesterol.
3. Eat five to nine servings of fruits and vegetables a day.
4. Help yourself to plenty of foods made with whole grains.
5. Keep calories under control.

> "In truth, the heart healthy diet is not about deprivation—it's about eating well."

✔ Choose leaner cuts of meat
✔ Remove fat from meat whenever possible
✔ Downsize your meat portions
✔ Add more beans and less meat to your favorite chili
✔ Substitute low-fat yogurt for sour cream
✔ Switch to a lower-fat milk
✔ Enjoy sherbet or nonfat frozen yogurt instead of ice cream

In this chapter, we'll show you how to turn that counsel into a satisfying way of eating that won't leave you hungry or longing for something forbidden. It isn't difficult. In fact, many of the world's most cherished traditional cuisines, from Italian pastas and Moroccan couscous to Chinese stir-fries and Mexican rice dishes, follow these simple precepts. Find out how delicious they can be!

Good Fat, Bad Fat

No wonder fat has a bad name. For one thing, it's very high in calories. Gram for gram, fat contains more than twice as many calories as carbohydrates. Worse, it's become synonymous with

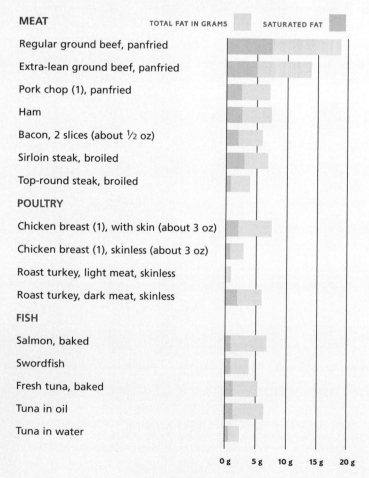

FATS IN MEAT, POULTRY, AND FISH

A serving size is 3 ounces unless otherwise indicated.

MEAT	TOTAL FAT IN GRAMS	SATURATED FAT
Regular ground beef, panfried		
Extra-lean ground beef, panfried		
Pork chop (1), panfried		
Ham		
Bacon, 2 slices (about ½ oz)		
Sirloin steak, broiled		
Top-round steak, broiled		
POULTRY		
Chicken breast (1), with skin (about 3 oz)		
Chicken breast (1), skinless (about 3 oz)		
Roast turkey, light meat, skinless		
Roast turkey, dark meat, skinless		
FISH		
Salmon, baked		
Swordfish		
Fresh tuna, baked		
Tuna in oil		
Tuna in water		

0 g   5 g   10 g   15 g   20 g

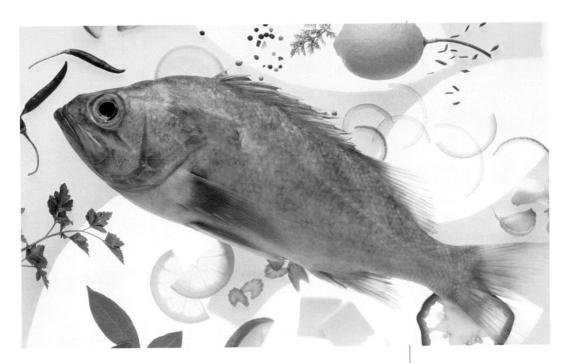

clogged arteries. For years, slashing fat has been considered job one when it comes to improving your diet.

But now we know that not all fat is created equal. Study after study has shown that one kind of fat is particularly dangerous to your arteries, and that's saturated fat, the kind found in meat, cheese, butter, and other high-fat dairy products. When researchers look at different diets around the world, they find that the higher the amount of saturated fat people consume, the higher the rate of heart disease.

Another kind of fat, the unsaturated variety, actually turns out to be beneficial to your heart. Unsaturated fat is found in vegetable oils, nuts, avocados, and olives. The more unsaturated fat the diet contains, the lower the risk of heart disease.

How can one fat be bad for you and another good? The answer has to do with what happens in your body after you consume them. Saturated fat triggers the production of artery-clogging LDL cholesterol. The more saturated fat you eat, the higher your LDL and total cholesterol numbers are likely to be. Unsaturated fat, on the other hand, keeps LDL levels down and boosts artery-friendly HDL cholesterol. Unsaturated fat has been shown to reduce the risk of erratic heartbeats. And it helps prevent blood clots, which can trigger heart attacks.

One way to distinguish saturated from unsaturated fat is to think about where each originates. Saturated fat is found mostly in animal foods: meat and high-fat dairy products. Unsaturated fat comes from plant foods. Another way is by looking. Saturated fat is solid at room temperature (think bacon grease or butter). Unsaturated fat is typically liquid (think vegetable oil).

When low-fat diets were first applauded, many nutritionists recommended replacing fats with carbohydrates. Suddenly all kinds of low-fat cookies and cakes and crackers crowded grocery-store shelves, and we loaded up on them.

RATE YOUR DIET

How healthy is your diet? Answer these 12 questions and circle the number to the right of your answer. When you're done, add up your score.

How many servings of fruit do you eat on a typical day?
(A serving is 1 apple, banana, orange, pear, or other fruit or ¾ cup of juice)
- 3 or more 2
- 1–2 1
- 0 0

How many servings of vegetables?
(A serving is 1 cup of raw leafy vegetables, ½ cup of other vegetables, or ¾ cup of vegetable juice)
- 3 or more 2
- 1–2 1
- 0 0

What kind of milk do you drink?
- Skim 3
- Soy 3
- 1 percent 2
- Don't drink milk 2
- 2 percent 1
- Whole 0

Which of the following do you use most often when cooking?
- Olive oil or canola oil 3
- Cholesterol-lowering margarine 3
- Other vegetable oils 2
- Soft margarine 1

- Stick margarine 0
- Butter 0
- Vegetable shortening 0

How often do you eat salmon or other fish during a typical week?
- 4 or more times 3
- 2–3 times 2
- Once 1
- Rarely or never eat fish 0

How often do you eat beef during a typical week, including hamburgers?
- Rarely or never 3
- 1–2 times 2
- 3–4 times 1
- 5 or more times 0

What kind of bread do you prefer?
- Whole grain (whole wheat or multi-grain) 3
- Don't eat bread 1
- White bread 0

How often do you eat eggs during a typical week?
- Rarely or never 3
- 1–2 times 2
- 3–4 times 1
- 5 or more times 0

That wasn't such a good idea. Very low-fat, high-carbohydrate diets, scientists have realized, have an unwanted effect on cholesterol. True, they lower total cholesterol levels. But they also lower HDL cholesterol, the good kind. In addition, they raise triglycerides, which have been shown to be a risk factor for heart disease. Dutch scientists demonstrated the dangers of slashing fat and boosting carbohydrates very clearly when they tested two different eating plans on 48 volunteers. Half the subjects consumed a low-

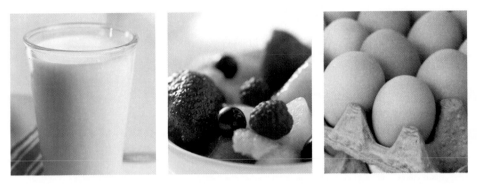

Which of the following foods do you eat frequently (at least twice a week)?
- Brown rice 3
- Whole grains like oats or barley 3
- Pasta 2
- White potatoes 0
- White rice 0

What do you typically have for dessert?
- Fruit 3
- Sherbet, ice milk, or frozen nonfat yogurt 2
- Don't eat dessert 2
- Cake, pie, cookies, or other pastries . 0
- Ice cream 0

What is your body mass index, or BMI (see chart on page 131)?
- 24 or below 3
- 25–29 1
- 30 or higher 0

Which of the following are you most likely to choose for a snack?
- Fruit 3
- Nuts 3
- Granola bar 2
- Pretzels 1
- Candy bar 0
- Potato chips 0
- Cookies 0

A score of 31 to 36 means you're already eating a heart smart diet. Keep up the good work, and you'll keep reaping the benefits.

A score of 23 to 30 means you've made some healthy choices. A few changes can help you lower your risk of heart disease even further.

A score of 0 to 22 means you have lots of room for improving your diet. This chapter will show you how.

Ways to Replace Saturated Fat With Unsaturated Fat

✔ Dip your bread in olive oil instead of using butter

✔ Cook with vegetable oil instead of butter or lard

✔ Use nuts or seeds in stir-fries instead of meat

✔ Add an avocado slice instead of cheese to your sandwich

✔ Try mayonnaise made with canola oil

✔ Pop popcorn with olive or canola oil and forgo the butter

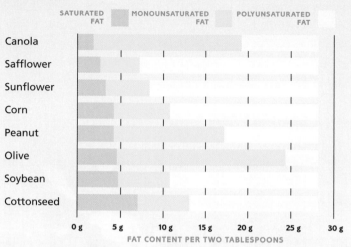

TIME FOR AN OIL CHANGE?

Oils with the most monounsaturated fat and the least saturated fat should be your first choice. Here's how common oils stack up.

TYPE OF OIL

	SATURATED FAT	MONOUNSATURATED FAT	POLYUNSATURATED FAT
Canola			
Safflower			
Sunflower			
Corn			
Peanut			
Olive			
Soybean			
Cottonseed			

0 g   5 g   10 g   15 g   20 g   25 g   30 g

FAT CONTENT PER TWO TABLESPOONS

fat, high-carbohydrate diet. The others ate foods low in saturated fat but rich in olive oil, an unsaturated fat. Total cholesterol levels fell in both groups. But among the volunteers on the low-fat, high-carb diet, HDL levels plummeted, and triglycerides soared.

Such results have convinced many heart experts that the best advice isn't to cut total fat but rather to replace saturated fat with unsaturated fat. That's great news if you love good food. Instead of butter, you can use olive or canola oil, both rich in unsaturated fat. In place of a plate of bland steamed vegetables, you can sauté your favorites—from carrots and broccoli to spinach and mustard greens—in savory olive oil. Instead of low-fat crackers, with all the taste of sawdust, you can reach for a handful of delicious dry-roasted nuts. And because fish is rich in unsaturated fat, you can serve up as much as you'd like. Fish oil, in fact, appears to be one of the heart healthiest oils around.

For proof, look at Eskimos. One of the favorite delicacies among Alaskan natives is muktuk—strips of whale skin and blubber. No wonder the Eskimo diet is sky-high in fat. Yet, Eskimos have a surprisingly low incidence of heart disease. The reason: Fish makes up a large part of their diet, and fish contains a form of unsaturated fat, called omega-3 fatty acid, that is believed to protect against heart disease.

Studies have shown that omega-3s lower triglyceride levels. They may also reduce the risk of small blood clots that can lead to heart attacks. Further, fish oil seems to stabilize the heartbeat, lowering the risk of irregular heart rhythms associated with sudden cardiac failure. In the Seven Countries Study, which looked at heart disease risk in different populations around the world, researchers found that men who ate no fish had the highest rate of death from coronary artery disease. Those who ate the most fish had the lowest rate.

How low should you go?

Experts agree that it's important to eat less saturated fat. But they disagree on how much total fat a healthy diet should contain. The American Heart Association and the National Cholesterol Education Program say fat calories should represent less than 30 percent of total calories. Saturated fat should account for no more than 10 percent of total calories.

Battle of the Omegas

Unsaturated oils come in two forms: monounsaturated and polyunsaturated. Olive oil is especially rich in the former. Corn oil and soybean oil are loaded with the latter. Which is the healthier choice? Both are good for your heart. Some experts suspect there may be an optimum balance between the two, but so far no one agrees on what that may be.

What may matter more, some researchers think, is the balance between two types of polyunsaturated fat. The first, found in vegetable oils like corn oil, is rich in omega-6 fatty acids. The second, found in fish, contains omega-3s. Flaxseed, walnuts, and canola oil are other good sources of omega-3s. Physician Artemis Simopoulos, who led the nutrition-coordinating committee of the National Institutes of Health for nine years, thinks most Americans should eat more omega-3 fatty acids and less omega-6. Why? According to Simopoulos, omega-3s block inflammatory diseases such as arthritis and colitis, while omega-6s may promote them. Omega-3s may also reduce the risk of cancer. One simple way to add omega-3s is to eat more fish and cook with canola oil (it has the advantage of having almost no flavor, so you can use it without affecting the taste of dishes).

But some researchers aren't convinced that it's worth worrying about balancing omega-3s and omega-6s. Nor do they think you need to bother about monounsaturated fat versus polyunsaturated fat. The real key is eating less saturated fat, both by consuming fewer foods loaded with saturated fat and by replacing saturated with unsaturated fat.

MEALS FOR ALL SEASONS

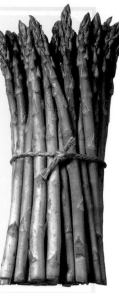

One of the joys of fruits and vegetables is their seasonality. Ripe pears come around only once a year. The most tender asparagus arrives in spring. Late summer brings luscious tomatoes. By November the markets are full of acorn squash and fresh cranberries.

Let the season's produce inspire your meals. When the first local tomatoes appear at farmer's markets, serve them sliced with olive oil and vinegar or roughly chopped in your favorite pasta. If you like spicy greens, make a salad with watercress or arugula. On a sultry summer day, cool yourself down with chilled gazpacho, a cold soup made with finely diced tomatoes, onions, green peppers, and parsley. Enjoy pumpkin bread in the fall and baked squash on a winter's night.

> "Replacing just 5 percent of saturated fat with unsaturated fat can reduce your risk of heart attack by about 40 percent."

Some researchers think that's way too much fat. University of California, San Francisco's Dean Ornish, M.D., for instance, is convinced that the best way to prevent heart attacks is to slash total fat to less than 10 percent of calories and virtually eliminate saturated fat. In his landmark Lifestyle Heart Trial, Dr. Ornish tested such an ultra-low-fat diet—one that all but banished oil, meat, and dairy products—in heart attack survivors. The findings showed that a very low-fat regimen, combined with exercise and stress reduction, could actually clear out arteries clogged with plaque, reversing heart disease.

But not everyone agrees that low fat is the way to go. In fact, some researchers believe the healthiest diet is one with as much as 40 percent of calories from fat—as long as it's unsaturated. The model is the Mediterranean diet. It's not low in total fat, but most of the fat comes from olive oil and seafood. And that, many scientists now think, makes all the difference in the world.

In fact, when researchers looked at data from the Nurses' Health Study, they found no link at all between total fat consumption and risk of heart disease or heart attack. What did matter was the kind of fat. Women who consumed more unsaturated fat were less likely to develop heart disease than women who consumed more saturated fat. Replacing just 5 percent of saturated fat with unsaturated, the researchers calculated—switching from butter to olive oil, for instance, and favoring fish over beef—can reduce your risk of heart attack by about 40 percent.

The Mediterranean model

Another study provided further evidence in favor of fats. The Lyon Diet Heart Study, conducted in France, looked at 605 men and women who had survived a first heart attack. Some were asked to follow a diet with about 30 percent of calories from fat. The others were put on a higher-fat Mediterranean diet rich in unsaturated fats. It included more bread, vegetables, fish, poultry, and fruit, less red meat, no cream, and a special margarine made with unsaturated oil containing omega-3 fatty acids (also found in fish). After two and a half years, the investigators were ordered to stop the trial. The reason: The risk of death among people on the Mediterranean diet was so much lower than the risk for people in the first group—about 70 percent less—that the ethics and safety committee wanted everyone to be offered the Mediterranean diet.

How much total fat should your diet include? If you've already been diagnosed with atherosclerosis or coronary artery disease, talk this question over with your doctor. If your HDL levels are lower than ideal, a diet higher in unsaturated fat may make sense. If you're trying to lose weight, you may fare better on a lower-fat diet. Either way, it's important to look for ways to reduce saturated fat. The American Heart Association recommends no more than 10 percent of calories from saturated fat. If you've been diagnosed with heart disease, you may want to lower saturated fat even further, to 7 percent of calories.

A hidden danger: trans fat

Not long ago, researchers discovered another kind of fat that poses a serious heart danger: hydrogenated fat, also called trans fat. Trans fat is a man-made concoction, first devised by food chemists more than a century ago. By tinkering with hydrogen molecules, they discovered that they could turn liquid vegetable oil into a solid. The result: a vegetable oil that could be used instead of butter or lard. The first margarine was born. Soon vegetable shortening took its place in almost every cook's cupboard. Hydrogenated fats also showed up in all kinds of snacks and processed foods. Unfortunately, it turns out that these fats are almost as hard on your arteries as saturated fat. They raise LDL cholesterol (the bad kind) and drag down HDL cholesterol (the good kind).

10 Top Sources of Omega-3s

1. Salmon
2. Lake trout
3. Anchovy
4. Bluefish
5. Herring
6. Tuna
7. Whitefish
8. Crab
9. Lobster
10. Shrimp

IN THE DAIRY CASE

Still drinking high-fat milk? Time to lighten up. The easiest approach is to switch to the next lower level of fat—from whole to 2 percent, for instance, or from 2 percent to 1 percent. It won't take long before lower-fat milk tastes as good as what you were drinking before. And by lowering the fat in the milk you drink, you'll also reduce both cholesterol and calories. If your milk has added protein or milk solids, the numbers may vary slightly.

TYPE OF MILK	TOTAL FAT PER CUP	SATURATED FAT	CHOLESTEROL	CALORIES
Whole (3.5%)	8.0 g	5.0 g	34.0 mg	149
Reduced fat (2%)	4.7 g	2.9 g	19.5 mg	122
Low fat (1%)	2.6 g	1.6 g	9.8 mg	102
Skim (nonfat)	0.4 g	0.3 g	4.9 mg	86

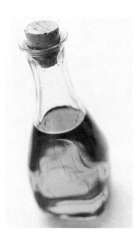

FAST FACT

When you're shopping for olive oil, choose extra virgin. According to Spanish researchers, this form, which is unrefined, is better than others at preventing the oxidation of LDL cholesterol that damages arteries.

Ridding your diet of trans fats isn't easy. They turn up in all kinds of foods, from margarines and vegetable shortenings to crackers, muffins, and cookies. The fast-food industry uses hydrogenated fats for deep-frying everything from chicken nuggets to french fries. How to avoid all this artery-clogging gunk? The Food and Drug Administration recently began requiring manufacturers to list hydrogenated (trans) fats on food labels, which makes it easy to identify processed foods high in these fats and avoid them. At fast-food restaurants, go easy on fried foods. And instead of snacking on potato chips, have a handful of nuts instead.

Whatever Happened to Cholesterol?

Remember when dietary cholesterol was public health enemy number one? When it seemed that all we had to do was buy foods marked "cholesterol free" and we'd never have to worry about heart disease again? Nutritionists say it's still a good idea to limit your intake of the stuff. But the obsession with dietary cholesterol has given way to a focus on saturated fat. Why?

For starters, the amount of cholesterol you consume isn't directly linked to cholesterol in your blood. When you eat cholesterol-rich foods, the cholesterol they contain ends up in your liver. There, it slows the liver's production of a protein that helps remove LDL cholesterol from the blood. So in theory, the more cholesterol you eat, the higher the level of LDL in your blood.

But in reality, the connection is a bit more complicated. The liver itself manufactures cholesterol, which is used to build cell walls, make hormones, and do other important tasks around the body. To keep blood-cholesterol levels steady, the liver keeps tabs on how much cholesterol is coming in from food. The more we consume, the less it churns out. That feedback mechanism helps keep cholesterol levels relatively stable.

Kinks in the process

In one out of five people, though, the feedback mechanism doesn't work. If you're one of them, it doesn't matter whether you eat a lot of cholesterol or a little: Your body goes on cranking out the same amount. In that case, minimizing the amount of cholesterol you consume is even more important, or else the combination of the cholesterol you get in food and the amount your liver produces will send your levels soaring. If your total cholesterol is above 240 mg/dL (milligrams per deciliter), chances are good your feedback mechanism may not be working right.

For most of us, researchers now say, it's much more useful to focus on cutting back on saturated fat. The more saturated fat you consume, the higher your blood-cholesterol level. Period. There's even a scientific formula: Each one percent decrease in calories from saturated fats in the diet produces a 3 mg/dL decrease in blood cholesterol. Focusing on saturated fat is useful for another reason: Many foods that are high in saturated fat—meat and high-fat dairy products—are also high in cholesterol.

Are eggs okay?

There are two main exceptions. Organ meats (liver and kidneys) and eggs are high in cholesterol but not saturated fat. Organ meats are so high in cholesterol that it's best to avoid them. As for eggs, you don't have to say no entirely, unless your cholesterol is in the stratosphere. But it's worth making them a special treat. Most experts recommend getting no more than 300 mg of cholesterol a day. If you've been diagnosed with atherosclerosis, your goal should be no more than 200 mg. One egg contains about 240 mg of cholesterol—enough to put some people over the top. So give eggs a break. But only now and then.

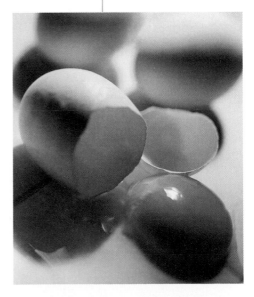

10 Foods Rich in Antioxidants

1. Spinach
2. Blueberries
3. Strawberries
4. Kale
5. Broccoli
6. Brussels sprouts
7. Cranberries
8. Prunes
9. Tea
10. Grape juice

The Rainbow Connection

How colorful is your diet? If it's bursting with greens, reds, yellows, and oranges, chances are you're eating the recommended five or more servings of fruits and vegetables a day. But most of us aren't. And that's too bad, because these foods are loaded with antioxidants—potent substances that fight cancer, head off heart disease, and protect against a variety of other chronic illnesses, from diabetes to macular degeneration. How? By blocking damage caused by unstable oxygen molecules known as free radicals. Such damage speeds up the process that turns artery-clogging cholesterol into potentially deadly plaques on vessel walls. Research suggests that oxidation is also the culprit in Alzheimer's disease.

The more fruits and vegetables you eat, the more protection you get. In fact, you'll find the richest array of antioxidants—from vitamin A to zeaxanthin—in the produce aisle. While the official advice is to eat between 5 and 9 servings of fruits and veggies a day, some research suggests the optimal number of these low-fat, high-fiber foods may be as great as 10.

Leafy green vegetables are also loaded with the B vitamin folate (the word comes from foliage). So are citrus fruits. Folate keeps homocysteine levels in the bloodstream from rising—and that can dramatically lower your risk of heart disease. If you've just had heart bypass surgery, one recent study found, plenty of folate in your diet can prevent arteries from reclogging.

A diet rich in fruits and vegetables can head off strokes as well as heart attacks, according to a 1999 report in the *Journal of the American Medical Association.* Scientists found that people who consumed around six servings of fruits and vegetables a day were 30 percent less likely to have a stroke during the 14-year investigation than those who rarely ate foods from the produce aisle. The greatest protection came from leafy green vegetables, cruciferous vegetables like broccoli and cauliflower, and citrus fruit and fruit juice—all abundant sources of fiber.

Fiber for your heart

Something all vegetables and fruits have in common is a load of fiber—that part of plant foods the body can't digest. Fiber comes in two basic types. The insoluble kind passes through the digestive tract unchanged. The soluble kind dissolves to form a gummy substance in the intestines.

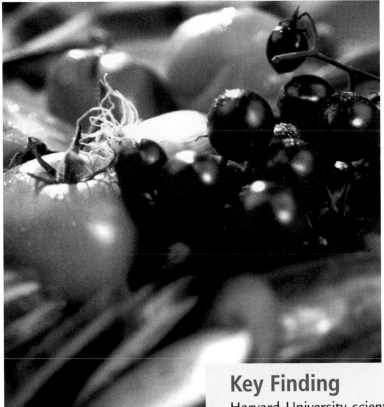

Key Finding

Harvard University scientists found that volunteers who consumed more than 24 grams of fiber a day were 50 percent less likely to develop high blood pressure than those who consumed less than 12 grams daily.

Both types are important to heart health. Here's why. Insoluble fiber slows the progress of food through the intestines, which helps keep blood-sugar and insulin levels from rising too fast. That, in turn, can lower your risk of type II diabetes and coronary artery disease. When soluble fiber turns gummy, it traps cholesterol and helps remove it from the body. Fiber also contains natural anticlotting agents, which can help prevent the small clots that trigger heart attacks and strokes.

There's plenty of evidence that helping yourself to foods rich in fiber offers powerful heart protection. In a 1999 study by researchers from Children's Hospital in Boston, men and women who consumed the greatest amount of fiber every day were found to have significantly lower blood pressure, triglyceride levels, and LDL cholesterol than those who ate the least. They were also less likely to gain weight. Among Caucasians, the fiber eaters averaged 167 pounds, compared with 175 pounds for the low-fiber group.

FAST FACT

Americans' daily intake of fiber has declined by a whopping 80 percent over the past century. One reason: Meats and fatty foods have crowded out vegetables, fruits, and whole-grain foods from our plates.

Foods High in Soluble Fiber

1. Oat bran
2. Beans
3. Peas
4. Rice bran
5. Barley
6. Citrus fruits
7. Strawberries

Foods High in Insoluble Fiber

1. Whole-wheat breads
2. Wheat cereals
3. Rice
4. Barley and other grains
5. Cabbage
6. Beets
7. Carrots
8. Brussels sprouts
9. Turnips
10. Cauliflower

Among African-Americans, the high-fiber group averaged 177 pounds compared with 185 pounds for the low-fiber group. Harvard University scientists recently found that women who ate the most fiber also had the lowest risk of diabetes.

Not yet convinced it's worth steering your cart to the produce aisle? Consider this: New findings from the Harvard School of Public Health show that every helping of fruit or vegetables you add to your daily menu cuts your heart disease risk by 4 percent. That may not sound like a lot. But the study, which followed more than 130,000 men and women over a period of 8 to 14 years, found that those who ate the most produce were 20 percent less likely to get coronary artery disease than those who ate the least.

Americans' daily intake of fiber has declined by a whopping 80 percent over the past century. One reason: Meats and fatty foods have crowded out vegetables, fruits, and whole-grain foods from our plates. If you have risk factors for heart disease—a family history of early heart attacks, for instance, or elevated cholesterol—it's especially well worth shooting for more than five servings of fruits and vegetables a day. Heck, why not set your sights on 10? Impossible, you say? Not at all. Here's what a day's meal plan might look like.

Breakfast
- 1 eight-ounce glass of orange or grapefruit juice
- Whole-grain cereal with raisins and banana slices or berries

Morning snack
- 1 apple or pear

Lunch
- Chicken or turkey sandwich on whole-grain bread with lettuce and tomato
- Coleslaw

Afternoon snack
- Carrot and celery sticks or a glass of tomato or V-8 juice

Dinner
- Tuna casserole with broccoli or corn
- Side dish of roasted beets or squash
- Leafy green salad

Dessert
- Mixed berries

Tally: 4 servings of fruit and 6 servings of vegetables, for a grand total of 10 servings.

Five Superstar Foods

Almost any food high in fiber, rich in antioxidants, or low in saturated fat is good for your heart. But some foods offer special benefits. Here are five worth stocking up on.

1. Nuts. Once banished from the list of healthy foods because of their high fat content, nuts are suddenly back. Studies show that eating more nuts could actually lower your heart disease risk. In the Nurses' Health Study, for instance, which followed more than 86,000 women from around the country, those who ate more than five ounces of nuts a day lowered their risk of a nonfatal heart attack by 32 percent, compared with women who didn't eat nuts. Plus the risk of a fatal heart attack was 39 percent lower.

Besides being rich in unsaturated fat, nuts also contain arginine, an amino acid that is needed to make nitric oxide. Nitric oxide in turn helps relax constricted blood vessels and increase blood flow. Nuts are also good sources of vitamin E, an antioxidant. Because nuts are high in calories, enjoy them in moderation, especially if you're trying to lose weight. Almonds and walnuts are especially heart healthy choices because the fat they contain is almost entirely unsaturated.

2. Lentils. One reason to love lentils is the fiber they contain. A single cup is packed with 16 grams of fiber—well over half the amount experts say we should be getting every day. In a study of 11,629 men and women enrolled in the Scottish Heart Health

FAST FACT

Cooking can damage or destroy some important disease-fighting substances, including vitamin C and folate. So try to eat a serving or two of fresh, uncooked vegetables and fruits every day.

WHAT'S IN A NUT?

Nuts are loaded with fat and sometimes salt. But they're no longer banned from a heart-healthy menu because the fat they contain is mostly unsaturated—so they're actually good for your heart.

NUT (1 OZ)	CALORIES	TOTAL FAT	SATURATED FAT
Almonds	167	15 g	1 g
Cashews	160	13 g	3 g
Macadamia	199	21 g	3 g
Peanuts	160	14 g	3 g
Pistachios	170	14 g	2 g
Walnuts	180	17 g	1 g
Mixed nuts (dry roasted)	180	14 g	2 g

REAL PEOPLE, REAL WISDOM

Heeding a Wake-up Call

The snacks were laid out. The Super Bowl party was about to begin. And suddenly William Shumacher, a San Francisco lawyer, realized he couldn't ignore the pain in his chest any longer. "I'd noticed it the night before. I figured it would go away on its own. But when it didn't, I suddenly thought, uh-oh."

An hour later, at the emergency room, Shumacher was being prepared for an angiogram. "I'd expected to be watching the Super Bowl," he remembers now, with a laugh. "Instead I found myself watching a television monitor that showed the catheter snaking through my arteries, injecting dye."

The test revealed a serious blockage of an artery supplying blood to his heart. Immediately doctors performed an angioplasty, opening the artery by inflating a balloon inside the blood vessel and then inserting a metal stent to keep it from closing up again.

Afterward, Shumacher realized that he was going to have to start exercising and change the way he ate if he wanted to avoid having a heart attack. "I was up to 215 pounds. And I pretty much ate whatever I wanted. Well, let me tell you, there's nothing like coming that close to having a heart attack to make you take all the advice you hear about exercise and diet seriously."

The first thing he did was install a treadmill and an exercise bike at home. Then he began paying attention to what he ate. "I gave up butter completely, just like that. And frankly, I never really missed it. I found myself enjoying the taste of bread for its own sake. I began to have fish when before I might have ordered a steak. I eat oatmeal now for breakfast instead of pastries. And when I go to a restaurant I look for dishes that I know will have a lot of vegetables in them, like Chinese stir-fries or vegetable soups."

It hasn't been easy for him to lose weight, though he is down about 15 pounds. Just as important, his blood pressure, which had been too high, is out of the danger zone. "The funny part is that I almost find myself enjoying eating more than I used to. I have to pay attention to what I eat now, which means I really take the time to savor it. I've discovered kinds of fish and vegetables that I didn't even know I liked. I'm eating differently. But I've never felt as if I've had to deny myself."

Study, researchers at the University of Reading looked for links between fiber, antioxidants, and cardiovascular disease. In women, fiber was the real standout. A high-fiber diet was found to cut heart-disease risk nearly in half. Lentils are also an abundant source of folic acid, which helps protect arteries by keeping blood levels of homocysteine in check.

3. Tea. Tea is steeped in a variety of potent antioxidants that help protect arteries from damage from free radicals, unstable oxygen molecules that make cholesterol more likely to stick to artery walls. A 1999 study found that women who drank a cup or two of black tea a day were 54 percent less likely to develop severe atherosclerosis than those who rarely drank tea. The more tea the women drank, the more they benefited. Those who poured four cups a day reduced their risk of atherosclerosis by 69 percent. Tea also inhibits blood clotting, which can lead to a heart attack or stroke. Green tea contains more protective antioxidants than black tea, although both have been shown to lower heart disease risk.

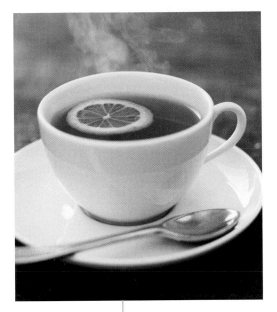

4. Soy. Not long ago the government gave food manufacturers the green light to promote the cholesterol-lowering benefits of soy foods such as tofu and soy nuts. A variety of studies have shown that people with elevated cholesterol who add 25 grams of soy protein to their daily menu can expect to lower total cholesterol by about 9 percent and LDL cholesterol, the artery-clogging kind, by as much as 15 percent.

And the benefits may go beyond cholesterol. In Japan and China, where soy is served at almost every meal, rates of breast cancer and prostate cancer are one-fourth what they are in the United States. No one knows for sure that soy is the reason, since Asian diets differ in many ways from ours. But when Japanese researchers compared 1,186 women with breast cancer to 23,163 healthy volunteers, they found that women free of the disease helped themselves to tofu much more often than those who developed breast cancer.

5. Avocados. Avocados are rich in monounsaturated oil, the same heart-friendly fat found in olive oil and nuts. Ounce for ounce, they also have more soluble fiber than any other fruit. Plus, food chemists recently discovered that avocados are spilling over in a plant sterol called beta-sitosterol, which helps prevent cholesterol from being absorbed through the intestines. That means less cholesterol makes its way into your bloodstream. Other fruits and vegetables contain beta-sitosterol, but avocados have more of it than any of them.

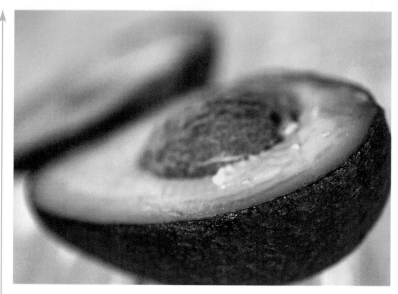

Ounce for ounce, avocados have more soluble fiber than any other fruit.

When researchers at Mexico's Instituto Mexicano del Seguro Social asked 45 volunteers to add avocados to their diets for a week, they recorded a significant drop in total cholesterol, artery-choking LDL cholesterol, and triglycerides. Volunteers in the study who had mildly elevated cholesterol saw the biggest benefit: an impressive 17 percent drop in total cholesterol and a 22 percent decline in LDL cholesterol. Because they're high in fat, avocados are also high in calories, so don't overdo it.

The Whole Truth

The more almost any food is processed, the less fiber and fewer nutrients it has—and the less protection it offers your heart. That's especially true of grains. Wheat in its unrefined state has an outer layer rich in fiber, magnesium, and vitamins. The germ at its center is a rich source of additional vitamins, including vitamin E, and unsaturated fats. Refined wheat flour (white flour), on the other hand, has been stripped of most of this goodness. The same is true of white rice (compared with brown rice, which still has its outer bran layer).

Key Finding

Protecting your heart may be as simple as eating the right breakfast. People who have a bowl of whole-grain cereal for breakfast every day reduce their odds of developing heart disease or having a heart attack by 37 percent, according to researchers at the Harvard School of Public Health.

A wild blood-sugar ride

There's another downside to highly processed grains. The carbohydrates in refined flour are much more easily digested and converted into glucose than the more complex carbohydrates in whole-wheat flour. The faster glucose enters the bloodstream, the steeper the rise in blood sugar. You may have heard in recent years about the glycemic index. A food's glycemic index number is determined by how much the food has been processed and how much fiber it contains, among other factors. Foods with a high glycemic index number (such as pancakes, cornflakes, and cooked potatoes) are converted into glucose much faster than those with a low number (such as bran cereal, pasta, apples, and skim milk).

A diet heavy with foods that rush glucose into the bloodstream can cause a roller-coaster effect. Here's how: The rise in blood sugar is followed by a parallel rise in insulin, the hormone produced by the pancreas that allows glucose to enter cells, removing it from the bloodstream. If glucose floods into the blood too quickly, the resulting spurt in insulin can drive blood-sugar levels too low. That dip triggers the body's hunger mechanism, which signals us to reach for something to eat. Grab something rich in simple carbohydrates, and you'll find yourself riding a roller coaster of blood-sugar levels throughout the day.

This wild ride, and the sharp hunger pangs that accompany it, can make it tough to maintain your weight. But there are more serious consequences. Spiking blood-sugar and insulin levels add to the risk of type II diabetes, which in turn increases your risk of heart disease—especially if you're overweight. Some researchers believe that the rise in highly processed foods in the American diet may be one of the chief causes of our epidemic of heart disease.

When researchers analyzed the eating habits of 75,000 women over the course of 10 years, they found that those who ate the most foods with a high glycemic index—white

To help keep your blood sugar steady, pour yourself a bowl of muesli or bran cereal instead of cornflakes.

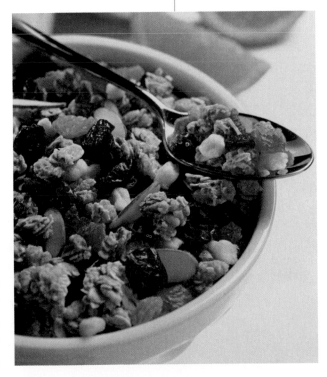

FAST FACT

One in five Americans eats less than one serving of whole-grain foods a day. Many barely have a single serving a week.

bread, white rice, potatoes, and low-fiber cereals—had an 85 percent greater risk of heart attack than those who ate the least. A surge of sugar into the bloodstream seems to reduce levels of good cholesterol, raise triglycerides, and interfere with the body's ability to use insulin.

Getting off the roller coaster

To avoid blood-sugar surges, opt for foods rich in whole grains and complex carbohydrates. In the process, you'll also take in more heart-protective fiber. And you'll get more nutrients and antioxidant vitamins with every bite. Here are a few simple tips.

- Start the day with whole-grain cereal. During the winter, sit down to a bowl of old-fashioned or steel-cut oatmeal (avoid quick and instant varieties, which are highly processed). For cold cereal, try GrapeNuts, WheatChex, Great Grains, Wheaties, and other brands that list whole wheat as one of the first ingredients.
- Opt for whole-grain bread. Look for packages that include whole wheat, whole oats, whole rye, or some other whole grain as the main ingredient on the label. Also check out the fiber content. Whole-grain foods typically contain plenty of fiber (at least 2 to 3 grams per serving). Highly refined ones usually don't.
- Try brown rice instead of white rice at dinner. Whole-wheat pasta and pizza shells are also showing up in more and more markets. When you cook, look for recipes that use whole-wheat flour—or at least allow you to substitute up to half of the white flour with whole wheat.

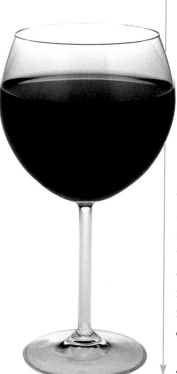

A Toast to Good Health

By all rights, the French diet should be a recipe for disaster. Goose- and duck-liver pates, creamy sauces, a whole course devoted just to cheese! But the French have some of the lowest rates of heart disease in the world. Why? No one knows the full answer yet. One reason the French may be able to get away with so many fatty foods is the fact that they typically consume more fruits and vegetables than Americans. Another may be their love affair with wine.

By now dozens of studies have shown that moderate consumption of alcohol offers some people real protection against heart disease. Men who drink one or two alcoholic drinks a day have 30 to 40 percent less risk of heart attack than men who don't drink at all. Women who imbibe an alcoholic drink a day also lower their risk of heart attack by about the same amount.

Alcoholic beverages bestow protection in several ways. For starters, drinking alcohol raises HDL cholesterol. It also reduces the risk of the kind of blood clots that can cause heart attacks and strokes. A recent study published in the *European Heart Journal* found that one of the most ancient of alcoholic beverages, wine, can open up arteries and increase blood flow.

Key Finding

The benefits of drinking wine may go beyond heart disease prevention. In a study published in 1998, researchers at Howard University Hospital, in Washington, DC, found that moderate wine drinkers are less likely than teetotalers to develop age-related macular degeneration, an eye condition that can cause blindness. Researchers suspect that the antioxidants in wine may protect against the damage inflicted by free radicals.

The downside of drinking

Despite the impressive evidence that moderate consumption of alcohol offers heart protection, many experts are reluctant to recommend that people who don't already drink start imbibing. For

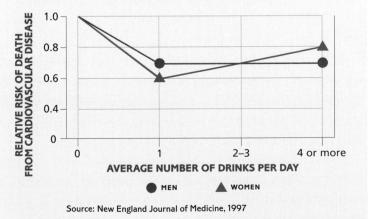

EFFECTS OF ALCOHOL ON RISK OF DEATH FROM CARDIOVASCULAR DISEASE

Research shows that moderate alcohol consumption lowers the risk of death from cardiovascular disease by up to 40 percent in people aged 35 to 69. Keep in mind that heavy drinking raises the risk of death from liver disease by as much as fivefold.

Source: New England Journal of Medicine, 1997

one thing, some people are susceptible to alcoholism. And excessive drinking can actually increase the danger of heart disease. It can also cause elevated blood pressure and heart-beat irregularities that can lead to blood clots. Too much alcohol can increase the risk of hemorrhagic stroke (the kind that involves a ruptured blood vessel in the brain). And of course, serious alcoholism can result in liver failure.

Even moderate drinking has raised some concerns. Several studies have shown that drinking two alcoholic beverages a day increases a woman's chance of developing breast cancer by 20 to 25 percent. Colon cancer rates also appear to be slightly higher in both men and women who drink. New findings suggest that the colon cancer culprit isn't alcohol itself but rather low levels of folic acid in the blood. Alcohol tends to reduce folic-acid levels. As a result, some leading nutritionists recommend that if you drink, you should be sure to take a multivitamin to keep your folic acid levels up.

Key Finding

Grape juice may provide some of the same protection you'll get in a glass of wine. Researchers at the University of Wisconsin Medical School in Madison asked 15 patients with clinical signs of cardiovascular disease, including narrowed arteries, to drink a tall glass of grape juice daily. After 14 days, tests showed a significant reduction in LDL oxidation, a crucial step in the formation of artery-clogging plaque. Ultrasound images showed changes in the artery walls, indicating that blood was flowing more freely.

The heart benefits that alcohol does provide don't apply to everyone. For men over 40, the merits of moderate drinking seem to outweigh any risks. But drinking offers little protection to people in their 20s and 30s, simply because their risk of heart disease is so low to begin with. In the Harvard Nurses' Health Study, the protective effect of alcohol didn't show up for women until after age 50. That makes sense, of course, since it's only after menopause that heart-disease danger climbs steeply in women. In men the benefits of drinking begin to show up after age 40. Even then, the people who stand to profit most are those with risk factors like elevated cholesterol or a family history of heart problems.

If you already drink, most experts say, make sure you don't overdo it. If you don't currently drink, don't feel compelled to start. You'll get just about the same heart benefits from increasing your level of physical activity.

A DASH of Prevention

Compelling new evidence tells us that just about everyone could benefit from eating a little less salt.

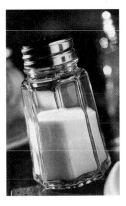

Should you cut back on salt in your diet? For years, experts have disagreed on the answer. Some studies showed that doing so helps reduce high blood pressure. Others found no benefit. Now a new study—one of the largest and most carefully designed investigations so far—says going light on salt really could help improve this leading risk factor for heart disease.

The new findings come from the Dietary Approaches to Stop Hypertension program, or DASH, sponsored by the National Institutes of Health. In a study of 412 adults, volunteers were assigned to eat either the typical American diet or the DASH diet, which is lower in fat and more abundant in fruits and vegetables, low-fat dairy foods, and whole grains, poultry, fish, and nuts. During the first four weeks volunteers in both groups consumed 3,300 milligrams of sodium per day—roughly the American average. For the next four weeks they cut back to 2,400 milligrams per day. In the final month they consumed only 1,500 milligrams of sodium daily.

The results were decisive. No matter whether people followed the DASH diet or the typical American diet, the less salt they consumed, the lower their blood pressure. The biggest benefit was in people with hypertension. But even people with normal blood pressure lowered their readings a few points by cutting back on salt. The biggest drop was seen when people followed the DASH diet with the lowest salt content.

Research shows that some people are more salt sensitive than others. Sensitive types are likely to get the biggest payoff by cutting back on salt. But the DASH results show that almost all of us can tame mild hypertension by going light on the stuff.

How? Shaking a little less on food is one way, of course. Instead of salt, try using pepper, lemon pepper, or other herbs or spices to add flavor. And instead of salty snacks like pretzels, reach for unsalted nuts, fruit, or carrot sticks.

To bring your salt intake down significantly, however, you'll have to look at the labels of prepared foods you eat. Many are loaded with salt. Consider this:

✶ One serving of leading canned beef ravioli in tomato and meat sauce contains 1,173 milligrams.

✶ A single serving of one popular frozen pepperoni pizza contains 1,022 milligrams.

✶ One brand of chicken-vegetable soup packs an astonishing 2,398 milligrams of sodium per can.

Fortunately, all processed foods are required to list milligrams of sodium on the label, so look for low-salt versions.

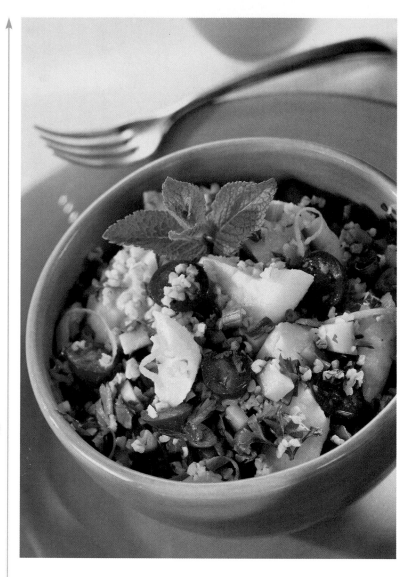

> If eating foods that contain protective substances is good for you, the thinking goes, taking a pill will be just as good. But is it?

Can't I Just Pop a Pill?

No sooner do researchers spot a substance in food that seems to fight disease than some clever entrepreneur begins to put it into pills or potions. Chances are your local health-food store is crowded with bottles containing all kinds of supplements, from vitamin E to multivitamins. If eating foods that contain these protective substances is good for you, the thinking goes, taking a pill will be just as good. But is it?

The evidence is still murky. People who fill up on fruits and vegetables loaded with the antioxidant beta carotene (such as carrots, mangoes, and yams) have lower risk of heart disease than people who get little—but beta-carotene pills have proved to have no benefit in several large studies. Worse yet, some volunteers taking beta carotene had a higher incidence of lung cancer.

Another antioxidant that has researchers scratching their heads is vitamin E. In a report that made headlines in 1993, women who took vitamin E supplements daily cut their heart disease by 30 percent. A study published three years later found that male heart patients who popped a daily E capsule were half as likely to have a second heart attack. Small wonder sales of the antioxidant quickly soared, making it one of the most popular pills on supplement-store shelves.

Then came the Heart Outcomes Prevention Evaluation study, or HOPE—the largest and most carefully designed investigation of vitamin E ever undertaken. The volunteers, including 2,545 women and 6,996 men, were all at high risk of heart attacks, either because they had cardiovascular disease or risk factors for it, such as diabetes. Half began taking a daily dose of 400 international units—the equivalent of 268 milligrams of vitamin E. The other half were given a placebo. Four and a half years into the study, the number of heart attacks, stroke, and deaths in both groups was precisely the same. Vitamin E hadn't offered any protection at all.

No one can explain these contradictory results. Some experts think a daily capsule of vitamin E may be powerful enough to prevent the artery damage that leads to coronary artery disease but not potent enough to reverse the disease once it sets in. Others think taking the pills is a waste of money, given the latest findings. Several large studies currently under way should help shed more light on the controversy. For now, the experts seem to agree, taking a capsule with 400 to 800 international units won't hurt you—and just might help prevent heart problems down the road.

Multiple benefits

Meanwhile, there is one supplement that it really does make sense to take: a multivitamin. Many Americans fall short on five essential vitamins: B_6, B_{12}, folate, D, and E. That shortfall can increase the risk not only of heart disease but also of cancer, infections, and even bone fractures. The best way to get all these nutrients is from foods, principally fruits, vegetables,

Key Finding

In a 2001 study at Tufts University, researchers found that older people who took a multivitamin for eight weeks had higher levels of B vitamins in their blood and lower levels of homocysteine—a substance linked to heart disease risk.

and whole grains. Taking a multivitamin isn't an alternative to filling your plate with nutrient-rich foods. But it provides extra insurance that you'll get the recommended amount, even on days when you can't eat quite as well as you should.

Recipe for Success

Good fat, bad fat. Complex carbs, simple carbs. Grams of salt and percentages of calories from fat. If you're feeling a little overwhelmed, relax. Healthy eating is really about making a smart choice each time you shop for groceries, sit down to order a meal, grab a snack, or plan your next dinner. And you don't have to make all the right choices all at once. Often it's easiest to develop more healthful eating habits meal by meal, day by day.

Often it's easiest to develop more healthful eating habits meal by meal, day by day.

Your first step: Pick one change you'd like to make. Then formulate a plan for how you'll do it. Finally, keep track so you know how well you're doing. Let's say your goal is to eat an extra serving or two of foods from the produce section. Decide on a specific strategy to make that happen—adding berries or bananas to your cereal in the morning and an extra vegetable dish at dinner, for instance. Keeping baby carrots in the fridge and making them your snack of choice. Or brown-bagging your lunch and including a piece of fresh fruit or a box of raisins and lettuce and tomato on your sandwich. For the next couple of weeks, keep an informal food diary of what you eat at each meal. If you fall short of your goal now and then, don't give up. Just try to do better tomorrow.

Here are 10 simple changes you can make that will help protect your heart. This week, check off two or three. Come back to the list after you've incorporated them and choose two more. Within a month, you will have gone most of the way toward adopting a heart smart diet.

1. If you drink milk, switch to a lower-fat variety.

2. Pour yourself a bowl of whole-grain cereal for breakfast at least three times a week.

3. Have fruit instead of your usual dessert at least three times a week. (Try baked apples or a fresh fruit salad.)

4. Switch from white bread to whole-grain bread.

5. Instead of dining on beef, choose fish, turkey, chicken, or a very lean cut of pork most days of the week.

6. Instead of ice cream, opt for sherbet, sorbet, ice milk, or nonfat frozen yogurt.

7. In place of potatoes or white rice, have whole-wheat pasta or brown rice at least once a week. Or experiment with grains you haven't tried before, such as barley or bulgur (cracked wheat).

8. Add one more serving of vegetables at dinner, either as a side dish or as part of the main meal. (Instead of pasta with meat sauce, for instance, opt for pasta primavera. Or try zucchini lasagna.) Stock your freezer with frozen veggies to help you meet your goal.

9. Put a bowl of fruit in a prominent place and help yourself when hunger hits.

10. Sauté foods in canola or olive oil instead of butter, margarine, or vegetable shortening.

Calories count

There is one last crucial component to heart smart eating: calorie balance. Being overweight or obese significantly increases the odds of developing heart disease—and nearly half of all Americans now fit into that category. The reason is simple: Too many of us take in more calories than we burn. If your body mass index, or BMI (see page 131), is in the healthy zone, you're doing fine. If your BMI is high, keeping an eye on the calories you consume is important. In Chapter Seven we'll take a closer look at losing weight and keeping it off.

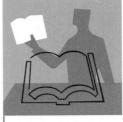

TERMS TO KNOW

ANTIOXIDANT A substance that neutralizes free radicals, unstable oxygen molecules that might otherwise damage healthy tissue

CARBOHYDRATE A chemical component of food that can take the form of sugars, starches, or cellulose

CHOLESTEROL (DIETARY) A waxy substance found in the fatty tissue of animals (no plant foods contain cholesterol)

GLYCEMIC INDEX A measure of how fast and how much different foods raise blood sugar

INSOLUBLE FIBER A form of fiber (found in whole grains, wheat bran, broccoli, carrots, asparagus, and pears) that is not fully broken down during digestion

MONOUNSATURATED FAT Heart healthy fatty acids abundant in olive, canola, and peanut oil

OMEGA-3 FATTY ACID A form of fat found in fish, certain vegetables, and seeds that protects against heart disease

POLYUNSATURATED FAT Heart healthy fatty acids abundant in corn, soy, and safflower oils

SATURATED FAT A form of fat (found mainly in meat and dairy products) shown to increase blood cholesterol levels. "Saturated" refers to the fact that every carbon atom is paired with a hydrogen atom

SOLUBLE FIBER A form of fiber (found mainly in citrus fruits, apples, potatoes, dried peas and beans, and oatmeal) that can be dissolved by the digestive tract

TRANS FAT Artificially produced fat created by adding hydrogen to unsaturated fat molecules, making it solid at room temperature. Trans fats have been shown to raise cholesterol levels

6

Getting Physical

Figuratively speaking, your heart is the wellspring of your emotions. But literally, it's a muscular organ, and muscles need regular workouts. If the only time you work up a sweat is when you worry, it's high time to fill the exercise prescription. You don't have to take up running or even join a gym. Studies show that even moderately intense activities—like brisk walking and ballroom dancing—will help you live longer and stay healthier.

Exercise not only keeps your heart strong, making it less susceptible to damage, it also helps maintain adequate blood flow to the heart and other parts of the body, keeping blood vessels in better shape. And that's just the beginning. When you give your muscles a workout, you make it easier for the cells throughout your body to process energy in the form of blood sugar, or glucose, which in turn helps lower the risk of diabetes, a serious risk factor for heart disease. Physical activity improves the ratio of good to bad cholesterol. Plus it reduces the risk of high blood pressure. People who are sedentary have a 30 percent greater chance of developing hypertension than people who are moderately active. And of course, burning more calories by getting off the couch helps you keep your weight under control, also crucial to the health of your heart.

Simply put, if a pill could provide as many benefits as exercise does, we'd all be clamoring to take it.

Public Health Enemy Number One

We all know exercise is good for us. Still, 60 percent of Americans fail to meet the official advice, which recommends at least 30 minutes of physical activity most days of the week. One in four of us, according to the latest statistics, gets no exercise at all.

It's easy to understand why we've become a nation of couch dwellers. These days we almost have to go out of our way to be active. Laborsaving devices have taken over most tasks that used to be done manually. Our lives are easier as a result. But we have far fewer opportunities to get our hearts beating and our lungs work-

> "If a pill could provide as many benefits as exercise does, we'd all be clamoring to take it."

Regular Exercise...

1. Lowers blood pressure
2. Boosts HDL levels and reduces total cholesterol
3. Increases strength and stamina
4. Expands lung capacity
5. Boosts the immune system
6. Builds muscle
7. Burns fat
8. Reduces the risk of diabetes
9. Protects against colon cancer
10. Eases depression and anxiety
11. Helps keep your weight in check
12. Maintains strong bones
13. Allows you to stay active as you get older

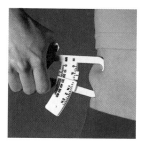

ing. According to one estimate, people in the year 1900 burned almost 1,500 more calories every day going about their business than we do today.

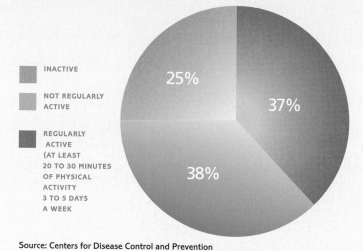

ACTIVITY LEVELS IN ADULTS

More than 60 percent of U.S. adults do not engage in the recommended amount of physical activity.

- INACTIVE
- NOT REGULARLY ACTIVE
- REGULARLY ACTIVE (AT LEAST 20 TO 30 MINUTES OF PHYSICAL ACTIVITY 3 TO 5 DAYS A WEEK

25%
37%
38%

Source: Centers for Disease Control and Prevention

Researchers are learning that being sedentary is more hazardous to your health than almost any other risk factor. A study from The Cooper Aerobics Research Institute, in Dallas, Texas, found lack of activity to be nearly as dangerous as smoking. Sitting around doing next to nothing is hard on almost every part of the body, from the bones to the muscles. But it's especially hard on your heart. According to the Framingham Heart Study, inactivity increases your risk of heart disease fivefold. Our bodies, in other words, are meant to move.

Are you healthy enough to exercise?

Most people, even those with heart disease, can safely get out and exercise. Still, it's smart to check with your doctor before embarking on a fitness program, especially if any of the following statements apply to you.

- I've been diagnosed with coronary artery disease or another heart-related condition
- I sometimes feel pain in my chest when I do physical activities or when I'm under emotional stress

- I'm worried that other health problems I have may worsen with physical activity

If any of these statements describe you, make an appointment to talk to your doctor before you begin a new exercise regimen—particularly one that involves moderately strenuous activities.

Your Exercise Prescription

Physical activities take two basic forms. The first, aerobic exercise, gets your heart beating faster and your lungs working harder. Examples include walking, jogging, dancing, swimming, and bicycling. You can tell an activity is aerobic if it leaves you feeling slightly or very winded.

The second, called resistance training or strength training, builds muscles, usually by making them lift, pull, push, or otherwise move something heavy. The classic way to strength-train is with weights in a gym. But you can also do simple exercises using portable dumbbells or even your own body weight.

Both forms are important for overall health. Strength training is especially key for maintaining what researchers call functional capacity—the ability to do what you like to do throughout most of your life, even when you are very old. Keeping your muscles in shape helps you keep your balance as you age. Strong muscles also help you maintain a healthy weight. The reason: Muscle tissue burns more calories than fat does, even when you're sitting still. Keeping your muscles strong also lowers the risk of type II diabetes by making muscle tissue better able to take in energy in the form of blood sugar.

But when it comes to your heart, aerobic exercise is more important. Researchers with the National Institute on Aging found that sedentary 60-year-old men who began

Key Finding

Adding moderate-intensity activity to your daily life increases the diameter of the arteries feeding the heart, which in turn boosts the amount of blood that reaches heart muscle. What's more, over time, new blood vessels begin to form, providing even more blood to the heart. Regular physical activity also increases the heart's efficiency. A study by researchers at the University of Leipzig in Germany found that exercise increased peak blood flow (the maximum amount of blood that can flow through arteries) by 200 percent.

Tips for Exercising Safely

✔ **Don't overdo it.** Gradually ease yourself into a new activity program

✔ Make sure you have a good pair of sneakers and comfortable clothes

✔ If you walk or jog at dusk or at night, wear reflective clothing

✔ If you ride a bike, wear a helmet

✔If you engage in sports that can involve falling, wear wrist and knee guards

✔ Drink 16 ounces of water before and after you exercise

✔ Stretch before and after you exercise (see page 106 for some basic stretches)

✔ Warm up by starting out slowly and gradually increasing the intensity level

✔ If you're exercising vigorously, cool down at the end with 5 to 10 minutes of slower activity

an aerobic-exercise program improved their lungs' ability to take in and deliver oxygen by almost 12 percent. The volunteers increased the amount of blood their hearts could pump by almost 10 percent. Finally, their hearts became more efficient, as measured by the percentage of blood leaving the heart during each heartbeat. All these improvements mean that more oxygen and nutrients reach all parts of the body, including the heart.

Tickle your fancy

Maybe you've put off exercising because you weren't sure how to begin. The first step is deciding what you'd like to do. Walk? Jog? Ride your bike? Swim? Join an aerobic-dance class? Take up a sport like tennis or racquetball?

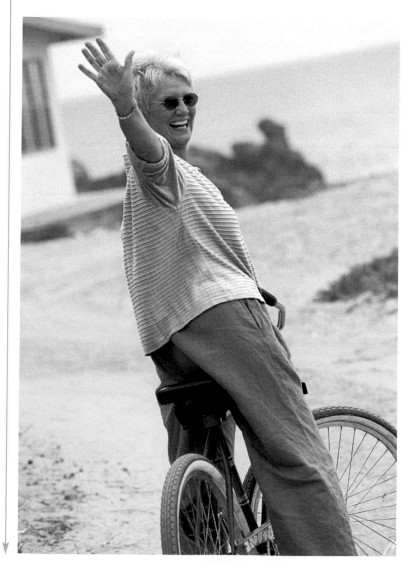

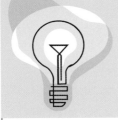

ASK THE EXPERT

How do I know if I'm exercising enough to help my heart?

Steven Blair, Ph.D., director of research at The Cooper Aerobics Research Institute, in Dallas, Texas, and senior scientific editor of the 1996 Surgeon General's Report on Physical Activity and Health:

"The good news is that you don't have to do athletic-style training to get most of the benefits of exercise. All you have to do is accumulate 30 minutes of at least moderate physical activity on most, preferably all, days of the week.

We're talking here about sedentary adults—people who aren't doing much of anything at the moment. If you're already more active than that, stick with what you're doing. But if you're among the 40 to 50 million Americans who aren't active, racking up 30 minutes most days will go a long way toward protecting your heart.

What do we mean by moderate activity? The most common example is walking briskly at between 3 to 4 miles per hour. To check your pace, map out a mile course in your neighborhood. Walk at your usual pace for a mile, checking your starting and stopping time. A brisk walk should take between 15 and 20 minutes. If yours takes longer, gradually increase the pace. Moderate-intensity exercise should leave you feeling winded but not gasping for air.

The official recommendations also mention accumulating 30 minutes. There was a time, 10 years ago, when exercise scientists thought you had to work out for a period of, say, 45 minutes to an hour to get heart benefits. Now we know smaller segments of activity can add up to the same benefit. Three 10-minute walks have the same payoff as one 30-minute walk. How short can an activity segment be? Are 30 one-minute walks the same as one 30-minute walk? The truth is, we don't know. No doubt there is a minimum duration. I suspect it may be around 5 or 6 minutes, but that's pure speculation. Still, if you've only got 5 minutes, it's better to spend it being active than sitting still. We sometimes encourage people to begin with 2-minute walks just to overcome the inertia that keeps many people sedentary.

Finally, we talk about most days of the week. I think it's smart to strive for 7 days a week, knowing that you're likely to miss a day here and there. If you accumulate 30 minutes of activity at least 5 days a week, you're doing fine.

Will you get more benefit by pushing yourself harder? Sure. But our studies have shown that if you go from doing nothing to accumulating 30 minutes of activity most days of the week, you'll cut your risk of prematurely dying in half. Do more than that—an hour of more strenuous activity— and you'll cut your risk by an additional 10 to 15 percent. The biggest payoff comes from moving out of the sedentary group into the moderately active group."

A BASIC STRETCHING ROUTINE

Stretching before exercise helps prevent injury. Stretching also keeps you flexible, making it easier to do many physical activities. Here are four simple stretches to get you started. Hold each stretch for 10 to 20 seconds. Repeat four times on each side.

■ Calf stretch

Stand several feet from a wall. Take a step forward with your left foot. Keeping your right leg straight and both heels on the ground, lean forward. You'll feel your Achilles tendon, at the back of your foot, and your calf muscles stretch.

■ Hamstring stretch

Sit on a carpet and stretch your left leg out in front of you without locking the knee. Bend the right leg as shown. Place your right hand on your left thigh for support. Bend over very slowly, keeping your back straight and your shoulders square, and reach toward your toes with your left hand. You should feel the stretch in the back of your thighs.

■ Quadriceps stretch

Place your right hand against a wall for balance. Grasp your left foot with your left hand and pull your foot gently toward your buttocks, keeping your standing leg slightly bent. Keep your left knee in line with the right. You should feel the muscle at the front of your thigh stretch.

■ Lower-back stretch

Lie on your back with your knees bent. Using both hands, pull your right knee to your chest, pressing your lower back into the floor. You should feel the stretch in your buttocks and lower back.

If you already know the answer, great. If not, think about the kinds of activities for which you are most likely to have the time and motivation. Some people prefer regular workouts at a gym. Others prefer activities like bicycling, dancing, hiking, or organized sports. A third option is to incorporate exercise into your daily life, by walking instead of driving, taking the stairs instead of the escalator, working in the garden, or throwing a Frisbee for the dog. Very active people usually combine several approaches.

What's right for you? Incorporating activities into your daily routine may be best if:

- You have trouble setting aside at least an hour three or four times a week to exercise
- You're uncomfortable with the way you look or embarrassed that you're out of shape
- You have a lot of chores around the house and garden to keep you busy
- You've just never been the gym-going type
- You enjoy walking

Joining a gym, YMCA, or fitness center may be the best option to choose if:

- You're motivated by having other people around
- You'd like to try classes in aerobic dance, yoga, Pilates, or other activities
- You would benefit from the help of a personal trainer or fitness expert
- You have bought exercise equipment before and watched it gather dust as it sits in the corner

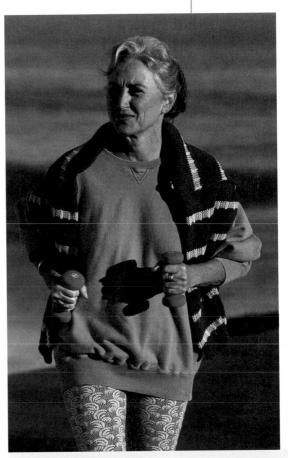

Key Finding

Moderate-intensity aerobic exercise could help you sidestep cold and flu bugs. According to a 1993 study, women who did a brisk 30-minute walk most days of the week reported half as many days with cold or flu symptoms than women who didn't walk. By increasing blood flow, researchers believe, exercise may boost the number of immune cells circulating through the bloodstream, enhancing the body's ability to detect and destroy invading viruses.

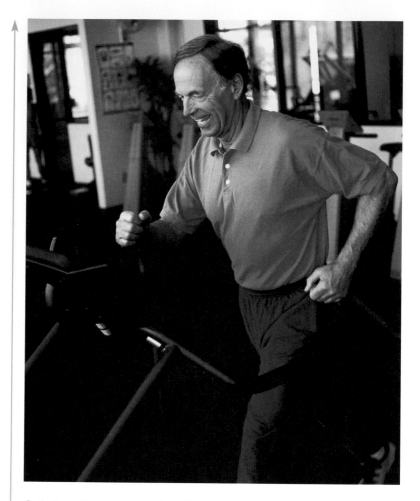

Joining the gym brigade

Millions of Americans stay active by joining local YMCAs, fitness centers, and other exercise facilities. There are many advantages to doing so. Most clubs have instructors who can show you how to use the equipment and create an appropriate workout program. Many offer classes in aerobic dance, water aerobics, yoga, spinning (using an exercise bike), kick-boxing, and other activities, as well as special programs for older people. The simple act of joining a gym can represent a big step in your commitment to exercise.

Before you sign up, however, make sure the facility is right for you. Too many people join with all the best intentions, only to let their membership lapse when they end up not going. Consider these questions before you plunk down money.

- Is the location convenient?
- Is the club well maintained and clean?
- Is the atmosphere comfortable?

- Does it offer everything you'd like (weight machines, pool, exercise classes, steam room, sauna)?
- Is the staff friendly and willing to help?
- Is the membership arrangement and price right?

Once you've chosen a health club, make an appointment to have an instructor teach you how to use all the equipment—even before you've decided what kind of exercises you'd like to do. You may discover that you love the cross-country-ski machine or the elliptical trainer, but you won't know until you try them.

Exercise "lite"

Not interested in joining a gym? No problem. You can get all the exercise you need by beefing up your everyday activities at home or around the neighborhood.

The notion that lifestyle exercise can offer all the benefits of full-blown workouts is sometimes called exercise lite. When experts first claimed that just 30 minutes of moderate-intensity activities could provide most of the benefits of more vigorous exercise, not everyone was convinced. So researchers at The Cooper Aerobics Research Institute decided to put exercise lite to the test. They recruited 235 sedentary men and women. Half

Moderate-Intensity Activities

1. Swimming
2. Bicycling
3. Cycling on a stationary bicycle
4. Mowing the grass (with a push mower)
5. Raking
6. Dancing
7. Walking briskly
8. Mopping or scrubbing the floor
9. Golf (without a cart)
10. Tennis (doubles)
11. Volleyball
12. Rowing

Vigorous-Intensity Activities

1. Aerobic dancing
2. Climbing stairs or hills
3. Shoveling snow
4. Tennis (singles)
5. Jogging
6. Hiking on hills
7. Downhill skiing
8. Cross-country skiing
9. Swimming laps

KEEP AN ACTIVITY LOG

The great advantage to lifestyle exercise is that you can do it whenever and wherever you happen to be. The challenge is making sure small bouts of activity add up to at least 30 minutes a day. The simplest way is to keep an activity log in a small notebook. Each time you take a brisk walk or climb the stairs, jot down what you did and how much time you spent. Just before dinner, tally up your activities for the day. If you've fallen shy of your 30 minutes, plan to take a brisk walk around the neighborhood after you eat. Here's what an activity log might look like:

TIME	ACTIVITY	DURATION
7:00 – 7:15	Walked before breakfast	15 minutes
8:00 – 8:05	Climbed stairs at work	05 minutes
12:30 – 12:45	Walked during lunch	15 minutes
5:30 – 5:45	Raked leaves in yard	15 minutes
TOTAL		50 minutes

agreed to do a standard gym-based exercise program, with treadmills, stair-climbing machines, stationary bikes, and all the rest. The others met once a week in small groups to talk about ways to incorporate physical activities into their daily lives, then followed through on their ideas.

At the end of two years, people in both groups had lowered their blood pressure by more than 3 points and lost the same amount of body fat (almost 2.5 percent). And all the participants were burning exactly the same number of calories.

The results convinced most experts that you really can create a heart healthy exercise program simply by looking for opportunities to get moving around the house and community. There are only three rules.

EASY WAYS TO ADD EXERCISE

Opportunities abound to add exercise to your everyday life. Here are some examples.

- Walking instead of driving to do errands within eight blocks
- Trading in your riding lawnmower for a push model if your lawn isn't too big
- Raking leaves instead of using a leaf blower
- Getting off the bus or subway one stop early and walking the rest of the way
- Parking at the far end of the parking lot and hoofing it
- Taking stairs instead of elevators and escalators
- Walking a full circuit around the mall or shopping center before you begin shopping
- Climbing stairs or walking during work breaks
- Volunteering for activities that keep you on the move (delivering meals to people in need, for instance)
- Walking the dog (if you don't have one, chances are a neighbor's dog would love the extra exercise)
- Riding a bike instead of driving whenever practical (be sure to wear a helmet)
- Joining a local hiking or biking club
- Taking a Western- or ballroom-dancing class

1. The activities must be at least moderately intense—vigorous enough to leave you feeling at least slightly winded (adding more vigorous activities is fine, of course).

2. You'll need to accumulate at least 30 minutes of activity most days of the week.

3. You'll need to keep track of how much activity you do.

Count your steps

If your activity of choice is walking or jogging, you can also use a clever gadget called a pedometer, or step counter, a small device that fastens to your belt or waistband and records each step you take. Step counters work by way of a small pendulum that swings each time you step. In The Cooper Aerobics Research Institute's landmark study of lifestyle exercise, step counters turned out to be extremely popular. Putting them on in the morning, participants were able to see exactly how many steps they took

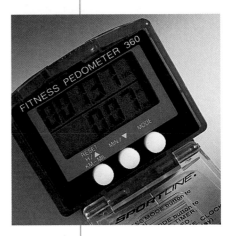

during the day. Many reported that the devices helped motivate them to exercise more. If the step counters showed they hadn't logged many steps by dinnertime, for instance, participants made a point of walking after the dishes were done.

Step counters, which cost between $15 and $35, are available at most sporting-goods stores. Shoot for 10,000 steps a day, and you'll do the equivalent of 30 minutes of activity. If you're trying to lose weight, raise your goal to 14,000 or 15,000 steps.

Two of the most reliable step counters are available by mail order. For information, contact New Lifestyles (888-748-5377 or on the web at www.digiwalker.com) or Accusplit (800-935-1996 or on the web at www.accusplit).

Walking Your Way to Better Health

Walking has become one of America's favorite forms of exercise. Small wonder. You can do it almost anywhere. You don't need to buy a membership card. In fact, the only equipment you need is a pair of comfortable shoes.

And even a short walk around the neighborhood can protect your heart from danger. When researchers at Brigham and Women's Hospital studied 72,488 nurses who were ages 40 to 65 at the start of the study, they found that those who walked the most

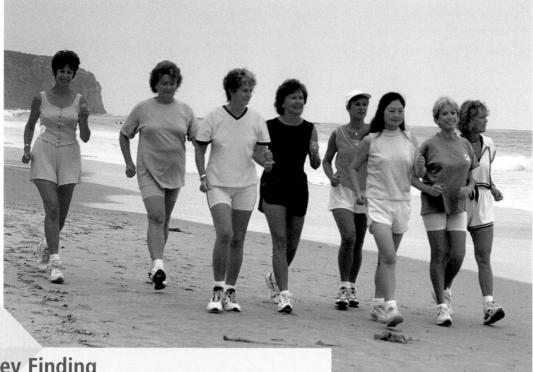

Key Finding

For women with diabetes, walking as little as four hours a week offers substantial protection from heart disease. In a study published in 2001, Harvard scientists found that those women who logged four to seven hours of exercise a week were half as likely to develop heart problems as women who rarely exercised. Walking was found to be just as beneficial as other, more vigorous, activities.

(three or more hours per week) cut their risk of coronary artery disease by 35 percent compared to those who rarely hit the pavement. Other studies have shown the same kind of protection for men.

Getting started

If you haven't done much walking, start slowly and gradually increase the time you spend and the distance you cover. Here's a monthlong program to start you off on the right foot. For safety's sake, always let someone know where you'll be walking and when you plan to be back.

Week One: Set a goal of walking at least 15 minutes a day, at least five days this week. Walk at whatever pace feels comfortable. Don't worry about the distance you walk.

Week Two: Increase the time you walk to at least 20 minutes. Push yourself a little harder—you should feel slightly winded without having to gasp for breath.

Week Three: Strive for a total of 30 minutes a day at least five days this week. Get into the habit of walking first thing in the morning and just before or after dinner.

Week Four: Walk 30 minutes at least four days this week. Try to keep your pace brisk. On another day set aside time for a 45-minute walk. To keep it interesting, plan to walk somewhere pleasant, like a local park.

Once you've built up to walking 30 minutes a day, you can get flexible with your walking routine. Take longer walks when you have the time. On busy days, break your walks into 5- or 10-minute chunks and try to accumulate two or three chunks.

Walking smart

A few simple tips can help you get the most out of walking and protect against injury.

Stretch first and last. Stretching before and after you walk will help you stay limber and avoid stiffness. See page 106 for four basic stretching exercises. Another good stretch for walkers is toe circles. To do these, stand on one foot, point the toes of your other foot and trace circles in the air, both clockwise and counterclockwise. Repeat with the other foot.

Start slowly. By gradually picking up your pace over the first minute or two, you'll get your heart and muscles primed before you hit your stride.

CHOOSING A WALKING SHOE

With more than 30 walking shoes on the market, buying the right pair can be a workout in itself. It needn't be. What matters most is comfort. If it feels good, chances are it provides enough cushion and support. When you're shopping for shoes:

■ **Try on both shoes.** Left and right feet are often slightly different in size. Find a pair that fits your larger foot.

■ **Wear the socks** you plan to exercise in. That way you'll make sure the fit is right.

■ **Allow a little extra room.** Your feet swell a little through the day, so buy sneakers with a thumb's-width worth of extra space between your longest toe and the end of the shoe. Make sure the overall fit is snug. If your heel slips or your foot can roll from side to side, the shoes are too loose and may cause blisters or even injury.

Walk tall. Keep your shoulders back and relaxed and your belly tucked in to protect your lower back. Keep your chin up to prevent strain on your neck. Your eyes should be focused ahead, not on the ground.

Find your stride. Walk steadily, letting your arms swing freely by your sides. The best rhythm and stride for you is the one that feels most comfortable and natural. If your strides are too long your head will bob up and down with each step.

Find soft surfaces. Concrete and asphalt are hard on knees and hips. A better bet: soft dirt roads, trails, or running tracks.

Listen to your body. If you feel pain in your joints or muscle stiffness, ease up a bit. If the pain continues, consult your doctor.

REAL PEOPLE, REAL WISDOM

For the Love of Walking

Ask Dolores York why she walks, and the first thing she'll say is, "Because I love it. I just love it." But there are other reasons. York's father died at 51 of a heart attack. "So the writing was on the wall for me to pay attention," she says. She'd also begun to worry about the weight she'd put on while she was raising two daughters, eating on the run, and being so busy she hardly had time to exercise.

So as soon as the girls were grown and out of the house, York hit the pavement. First thing in the morning or after she gets home from work, she walks through her neighborhood in New Canaan, Connecticut, covering three and a half to five miles most days. "One of the great things about walking is you can do it anywhere, anytime, rain or shine."

Something else she loves about walking is the way it keeps her in touch with community. "I moved to New Canaan about two years ago and didn't know anyone. By walking, I've gotten to know people around the neighborhood. That's very important to me."

These days York has a friend who often joins her on the walking circuit. "I'll call her, or she'll call me, and we'll agree to meet at the fire station in fifteen minutes. We chat nonstop. And I've noticed that when we walk together, we walk longer and at a faster pace."

Six months after beginning her walking regimen, York had lost 30 pounds. She's never felt better in her life. And if her daughters are right, she's never looked better. "A month ago they were looking at old photos, and they said, 'Gee, mom, you've gotten so hip looking. You used to be so dowdy.' I was 30 pounds heavier then, and I did look dowdy. When you exercise, you just feel better about yourself. You feel more comfortable in nice clothes. You carry yourself with more confidence. Whatever the reason, that's another big plus for walking," York says with a laugh. "I've become hip."

Add slowly. As you gain confidence and fitness, increase the speed or duration of your walks. To avoid strains, add no more than 10 percent a week to the time you spend on each walk.

Looking at Home Exercise Equipment

If you have a little extra room and a little extra cash, you can set up your very own fitness center at home. A University of Pittsburgh study suggests it's well worth the money for some people. The scientists enlisted 148 overweight women and divided them into three groups. Women in the first group walked 40 minutes at a shot, five days a week. Those in the second group walked 10 minutes at a time, for a total of 40 minutes. The third group also did 10-minute segments but with a crucial difference: The research team loaned them treadmills to use at home. Eighteen months later, the treadmill group had lost over 16 pounds. The women in the other two groups had lost between 8 and 13 pounds. These results suggest that people who have a treadmill end up getting more exercise.

You don't necessarily need fancy equipment, of course. If you decide to exercise at home, you can put together a simple home fitness center with nothing more than an exercise mat (for sit-ups and stretching exercises), a small set of dumbbells (for strengthening exercises), and a jump rope or an exercise video (for aerobic exercise). Then if you find you really enjoy working out at home, you can treat yourself to a stair machine or treadmill.

Before you buy anything, however, be sure you'll use it. Too many of us spend money on home exercise equipment only to see it gather dust. Before you spend your hard-earned cash:

1. Make sure there's a comfortable place in your house. If working out means going into a damp basement or dusty garage

Key Finding

Making any lasting change takes effort and commitment. Along the way, it's important to reward yourself for a job well done. Think of something fun you can do for yourself when you meet your weekly exercise goal—a dinner at your favorite restaurant, for instance, or new workout clothes. In a study at Brown University, researchers found that people who used rewards as a way to motivate themselves were almost twice as likely to stay active than those who didn't.

EASY AT-HOME MUSCLE TONING

These six simple exercises require nothing more than a little bit of room and a carpet or exercise mat. You can do them at home or when you're traveling. If you're exercising for the first time in a while, go easy—especially if you have back problems. Do as many repetitions as you can comfortably manage. A 20-minute session three times a week is all you'll need for good overall muscle toning.

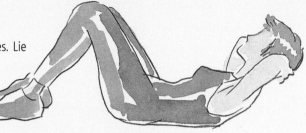

■ Sit-ups

These help tighten the abdominal muscles. Lie on your back with your knees bent and your feet flat on the floor. Keep the small of your back pressed against the floor. With your hands behind your head, fingers touching, and elbows pointing out, curl your upper body about a quarter of the way toward your knees. Use your abdominal muscles to accomplish this; do not pull on your neck. Hold for a "one Mississippi" count, then lower yourself back to the floor.

■ Push-ups

This classic is one of the best upper-body-strength exercises around. Lie facedown. Place your hands on the floor, pointing forward, directly under your shoulders, with your feet flexed. Straighten your arms as you push your body off the floor. Then lower yourself back down until your nose almost touches the floor, keeping your elbows by your body. To make this exercise easier, push off from your knees instead of your toes.

■ Squats

These target the quadriceps muscles at the front of the thighs. Stand with your legs about shoulder-width apart. Slowly lower yourself as if you were sitting on a chair—and just about as far—keeping your back straight and leading with your buttocks. Don't let your knees extend past your toes. Then raise yourself up again.

■ Arm circles

These will tone your arms, shoulders, and chest muscles. Extend your arms outward, as if you were preparing to fly. Then make small, slow circles with them, about as big around as a dinner plate. When your arms begin to tire, reverse the direction of your circles.

■ Skating in place

Here's a great workout for your lower back, buttocks, and hamstrings. Stand with your legs about a foot apart. Holding your arms out to the sides, shift your weight to your left foot and slowly lift your right foot, extending it backward at a 45-degree angle, knee slightly bent. Imagine you're an ice skater, and you'll get the feel of this exercise. Hold the position for a count of "one-two-three-Mississippi," then switch legs.

■ Dry swimming

This is a great exercise for lower-back muscles. Lie on your stomach with your arms extended in front of you. Place a rolled-up towel under your stomach to support your lower back, and one under your forehead. Tightening your buttocks and keeping your hips on the floor, simultaneously lift your right arm and left leg. Hold briefly, then slowly return to your resting position. Repeat with the opposite arm and leg. Shoot for a dozen repetitions.

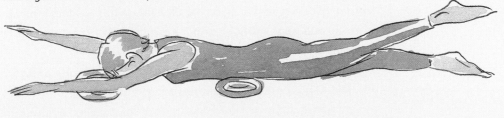

to use your exercise equipment, chances are you'll find a dozen reasons not to do it.

2. Check out rental options. Renting is a good way to try out different machines and see how faithful you are at using them before you buy. Some sports stores rent treadmills, stair-climbing machines, rowing machines, and other exercise equipment.

3. Evaluate carefully before you buy. Visit several stores before you plunk down money. Ask what features different models offer. And be sure to try a piece of equipment to see how it feels.

4. Ask about a maintenance agreement. Some equipment, such as treadmills and stair-climbing machines, need frequent adjustment and repair. Having a maintenance agreement could help guarantee that when a piece of equipment breaks down, you get it fixed and back on track fast.

Your Plan of Action

Whether you've decided to enroll at a gym, join a sports team, or add more physical activity to your everyday life, it's important to write up a plan of action. After all, it's one thing to tell yourself that you're going to become more physically active; it's another actually to do it. And the best way to make any change in your life, experts say, is to have a plan. Your action plan should include:

- A list of the kinds of physical activities you intend to do
- A schedule for exactly when and how long you will engage in these activities
- Your activity starting date
- How you plan to keep track of the amount of activity you do

Once you've drawn up your action plan, schedule your activities on your calendar for the next four weeks. Write down everything you intend to do: workouts at the gym, 15-minute walks during lunch hour, jogging with the dog. Then tell at least one family member and one friend about your resolution to become more active. Get in the habit of checking your calendar in the morning and again in the evening. Keep track of the activities that you completed and those you didn't get to.

During the coming month, don't worry if you miss a day or two. It doesn't mean your resolution has crumbled. It only means you've missed a day or two. Look back at your calendar, check to see what you've scheduled for tomorrow, and get back on track.

FAST FACT

A Finnish study recently found that fit men and women were two to five times less likely to die of coronary artery disease than people who were physically unfit.

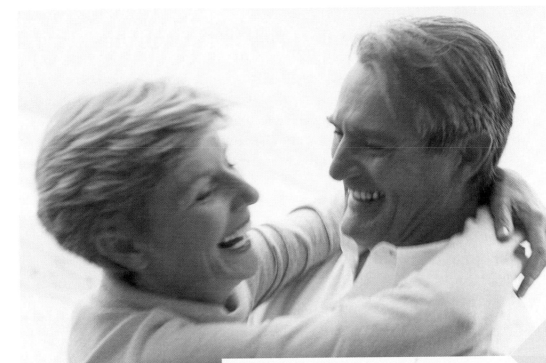

Key Finding

Older adults who participate in exercise programs are not only healthier but also happier, according to research by exercise scientist Kelli F. Koltyn of the University of Wisconsin at Madison. Koltyn studied 60 women older than 60 who were either living independently or in assisted-living communities. Those who were the most physically active rated their quality of life higher than those who were inactive, no matter where they lived.

Charting your progress

Once you have started your heart healthy activity program, chances are you'll want to know you're making progress. The fact is, simply by getting up and doing something when otherwise you would have been sitting around, you've made headway. Here are some of the benefits you may reap.

More stamina. Exercise scientists measure fitness by how long someone can walk or run on a treadmill. Fancy equipment can also measure how much oxygen the lungs can take in during strenuous exercise. But the simplest gauge is whether you can do activities like brisk walking or jogging for longer than before or whether you're able to increase the intensity of your activities—riding a bike up steeper hills, for instance, or walking a mile in 18 minutes instead of 20. If so, you're increasing your fitness level.

Lower blood pressure. Many people with hypertension who become more active see a drop in their blood-pressure readings

What's the Best Way to Measure Intensity?

Back in the days when exercise gurus thought you had to do strenuous activities to reap the health benefits of exercise, the usual way to gauge exercise intensity was measuring heart rate. The goal was to work out hard enough to get your heart rate into a certain range—your target heart rate (see below left). But some experts aren't sure that heart rate is a smart or even a safe yardstick, especially if you're over age 50. Medical conditions and certain prescription medications can affect how fast your heart beats. Beta-blockers, for instance, tend to keep your heart rate slower. Arrhythmias, or irregular heart beats, can also affect heart rate.

Using a target heart rate as your guide is controversial for another reason. The latest evidence suggests that you don't need to get your heart rate high to gain benefits. A better measure, many experts say, is the Borg Perceived Exertion Scale, which scores how difficult a particular activity feels to the person doing it (see below right).

In the end, the best method depends on how fit you are now and your exercise goal. If you're already active and want to increase your level of fitness, the target heart rate approach will give you the most accurate idea of how hard you're working your heart and lungs (provided you don't have a medical condition or take drugs that affect your heart rate). If you're just beginning an exercise program and your goal is to be active enough to protect your heart, the Borg scale is your best choice.

THE TARGET HEART RATE

Your heart rate is an indication of how hard you're working. The more intense your workout, the faster your heart has to beat in order to provide enough oxygenated blood to muscles. Target heart rate—the pulse you're aiming for during vigorous exercise—varies with age. See the numbers below. If you're taking high blood pressure medication, your target heart rate might be lower; check with your doctor.

Age	Target Heart Rate
30	95–142
40	90–135
50	86–127
60	80–120
70	75–113
80	70–105

THE BORG PERCEIVED EXERTION SCALE

Use this scale to describe how much you feel you're exerting yourself—from not at all to very, very hard. A score of 13 to 15, the "somewhat hard" to "hard" category, should put you roughly at your target heart rate. If your score falls below 10, try to push yourself a little harder. If your perceived exertion is above 17, ease back a bit to make sure you're not overdoing it.

6—No exertion at all
7—Very, very light
8
9—Very light
10
11—Light
12
13—Somewhat hard
14
15—Hard
16
17—Very hard
18
19—Very, very hard
20—Maximal exertion

over time. According to the National Institutes of Health, aerobic exercise reduces resting blood pressure in people who have hypertension by an average of 11 points off the top number and 9 points off the bottom one. For many people, that's enough to bring the numbers down into the safety zone.

Improved cholesterol ratio. Exercise often lowers LDL (the bad cholesterol) slightly, but its biggest benefit is increasing HDL, or good cholesterol. In one study conducted at Stanford University, volunteers who began walking or jogging 9 miles a week saw their HDL levels climb 13 percent.

Lower resting heart rate. Regular exercise makes your heart and lungs work more efficiently. That often means your heart will beat more slowly as you stick with your new activity regimen. A lower resting heart rate is a sign of cardiovascular health.

Weight loss. What most people hope for when they begin an exercise program is to lose a few pounds—and if you're overweight, chances are you will. But be patient. Losing weight through exercise is a slow process. The reason: When you exercise, you exchange fat for muscle. And muscle tissue weighs more than fat because it is denser. So the numbers on the scale may not budge right away. But you will be improving your body composition—and looking better in the mirror. And because muscle burns more calories than fat, increasing your muscle mass also boosts your metabolism. So over time, getting fit will help you maintain a healthier weight.

More self-confidence. Especially if you've been sedentary, becoming active is likely to boost your confidence level. You'll look better and feel better. And if you master an activity or two that you couldn't do before—aerobic dance or strength-training exercises, for instance—you'll enjoy a sense of accomplishment.

Overcoming obstacles

If you're like most people, your best-laid plans of becoming more active will bump up against obstacles—like a rocky period at work or a spell of foul weather that foils your daily walk. Sickness, holidays, even just a garden-variety bad mood, can make it hard to

TROUBLESHOOTING TIP

Not seeing the progress you hoped for? Don't be discouraged. Not everyone benefits in the same way from exercise. Some people lower their blood pressure dramatically; others see barely a drop. Some lose a lot of weight; others barely shed a pound. But whether or not you're making measurable changes, you're strengthening your heart and lowering your risk of a heart attack. In a study of 21,925 men, researchers discovered that volunteers who were obese but physically fit—measured by performance on a treadmill test—were less likely to die from heart disease than slim men who were unfit.

keep to your resolution. But for every obstacle, there's a way around it. For example:

When the weather turns frightful. There are plenty of opportunities to exercise indoors. You can walk in the shopping mall or at the local gym if there's a track. Or rent an exercise video.

WHAT'S IT WORTH?

Here are the number of calories you can expect to burn doing various activities. Of course, these are only averages. For more activities, log onto www.caloriecontrol.org/exercalc.html.

ACTIVITY	ESTIMATED CALORIES BURNED PER MINUTE OF ACTIVITY			
	120-LB PERSON	160-LB PERSON	200-LB PERSON	240-LB PERSON
Walking, 30-minute mile	2.4 calories	3.2 calories	4 calories	4.8 calories
Bowling	2.9	3.8	4.8	5.7
Dancing (waltz, fox-trot, samba)	2.9	3.8	4.8	5.7
Mopping, vacuuming	3.4	4.5	5.6	6.1
Bicycling, 10 miles an hour	3.9	5.1	6.4	7.6
Water aerobics	3.9	5.1	6.4	7.6
Weeding or digging in the garden	4.3	5.7	7.2	7.9
Aerobic dance, low impact	4.8	6.4	8.0	9.5
Playing softball	4.8	6.4	8.0	9.5
Walking, 15-minute mile	4.8	6.4	8.0	9.5
Playing tennis (doubles)	5.8	7.7	9.6	11.4
Horseback riding (trot)	6.3	8.3	10.4	12.4
Swimming laps (moderate effort)	6.7	8.9	11.1	13.4

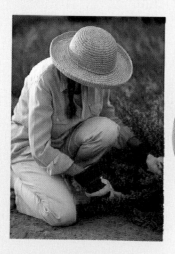
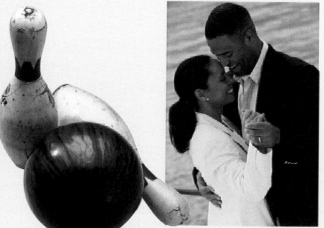

When work gets hectic. Remember that exercise can be a terrific antidote to stress. Taking just a 10-minute break for a brisk walk will clear your head and give you new energy to tackle problems. Or you might choose to get up a little earlier and exercise before work. That way, no matter what the day brings, your workout won't get squeezed out of your schedule.

If the people around you get in the way. Friends and family should encourage you to become more active. But that isn't always the case. Some people close to you may feel threatened by your new resolve to exercise. Some may even try to sabotage your efforts. If that's the case, sit down and talk about why becoming more active is so important to you. If appropriate, encourage family or friends to join you.

When the holidays hit. Make physical activity a priority by scheduling it on your calendar. If you have relatives visiting, explain to them beforehand that you'll be taking time out to exercise. You can also incorporate exercise into family activities, by ice skating, hiking, or walking on the beach together.

If you're feeling down. A case of the blues can make it hard to have the energy to do anything. That's the time to remind yourself that physical exertion can lift your spirits by triggering the release of mood-elevating hormones called endorphins. Some studies show it can even ease symptoms of full-fledged depression. If you just can't rally your spirits for your normal workout, at least go for a walk in a place you enjoy. You may find that getting up and doing something makes it easier to return to your exercise routine.

Moving forward

After the first month, take time to see how well your action plan is working. If you've kept an activity log, look it over. Use the quiz on page 125 to evaluate your progress.

If you're satisfied with what you did the first month, think about pushing yourself a little harder. The more active you are, after all, the healthier you'll be. If your goal is to lose weight, beefing up your exercise routine is especially important. The longer you engage in physical activities, and the more intense the activity, the more calories you burn.

When the second month is over, reevaluate your action plan one more time. If you're feeling a little bored with what you're doing, try a few new activities. Chances are your community offers all kinds of opportunities to get moving.

Join the Club

Many communities offer an array of clubs and classes to help get you in the exercise groove. Look for:

1. Bicycling clubs
2. Golf leagues
3. Walking clubs
4. Running clubs
5. Nature walks
6. Volleyball leagues
7. Softball leagues
8. Rowing and canoeing clubs
9. Water-aerobics classes
10. Tennis leagues
11. In-line skating clubs
12. Ski clubs
13. Ballroom- and Western-dancing classes
14. Environmental activities, such as beach cleanups

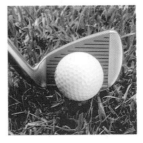

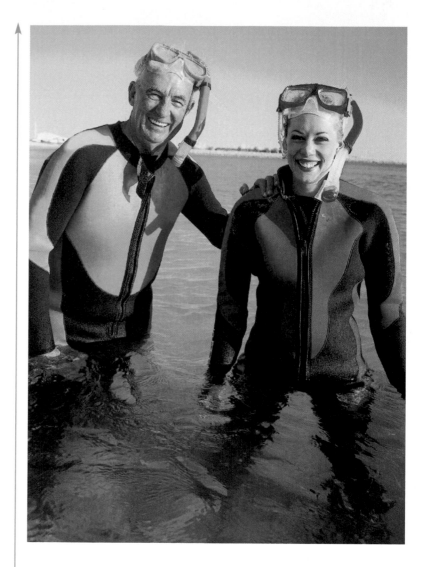

Remember, too, that no one is perfect. Chances are you'll go through periods when you aren't as active as you'd like to be. Now and then, you may tumble off the exercise bandwagon entirely. The worst thing you can do is decide you've failed and abandon your plan. If you falter along the way, get up, dust yourself off, and start again. Over time, physical activity may well become one of the best parts of your life—your chance to do something good for your heart, body, and spirit. Sign up for a bicycle, walking, or kayaking tour, and it could even take you to exciting new places. Imagine the possibilities!

TROUBLESHOOTING TIP

Need a little encouragement to reach your activity goal? The American Heart Association and The Cooper Aerobics Research Institute have created a nifty online program called Choose to Move, which lets you tailor a 12-week exercise regimen to your own goals and requirements. For information, call 1-888-MYHEART or log onto www.choosetomove.org.

HOW AM I DOING?

1. During the last month, I met my activity goals:
- Every day
- Most days
- Half the time
- Less than half the time
- Seldom or not at all

2. The biggest obstacle for me was:
- Not enough time
- Feeling down
- Trouble at home
- Getting bored with one activity
- Stress at work
- Other_____

3. What I like best about being active is:
- The chance to take a break from work to get up and move
- Spending time with other people
- Getting out in the neighborhood
- Feeling that I'm doing something good for myself
- Gaining confidence
- Other_____

4. What I dislike about being active is:
- Having to force myself to do something I don't feel like doing
- Taking time out from a busy schedule
- Working hard and not seeing the results I wanted
- Having to exercise on my own
- Feeling self-conscious about how I look
- Other_____

5. The most powerful motivator for me is:
- Setting a goal and sticking with it
- Putting exercise times on the calendar
- Exercising with someone else
- Rewarding myself with something fun
- Other_____

6. I would come closer to meeting my goals if:
- I had someone to exercise with
- I had more time
- I enjoyed what I was doing more
- My friends were more encouraging
- My schedule was less hectic
- Other_____

Not meeting your goals? Look back at your answers to fine-tune your action plan.

Item 2: Think of creative ways around your obstacles. If you're bored with walking, add a different activity, like bike riding or swimming.

Item 3: Write down other benefits you're getting. Post the list on the refrigerator. When you're tempted to skip your scheduled activity for the day, look at it.

Item 4: Brainstorm ways to take the bother out of exercising. If you're self-conscious about the way you look while exercising, rent exercise videos or consider buying a treadmill for your home. Or treat yourself to spiffy new workout clothes. If you dislike working out alone, sign up for an exercise class.

Item 5: Find ways to get even more leverage out of the things that work best for you. If setting goals really helps, make yours as specific as possible.

Item 6: Turn at least one item on your wish list into reality. If you wish you had more time, identify an activity that you're willing to forego. If you don't enjoy what you're doing, try out other activities until you find one you like.

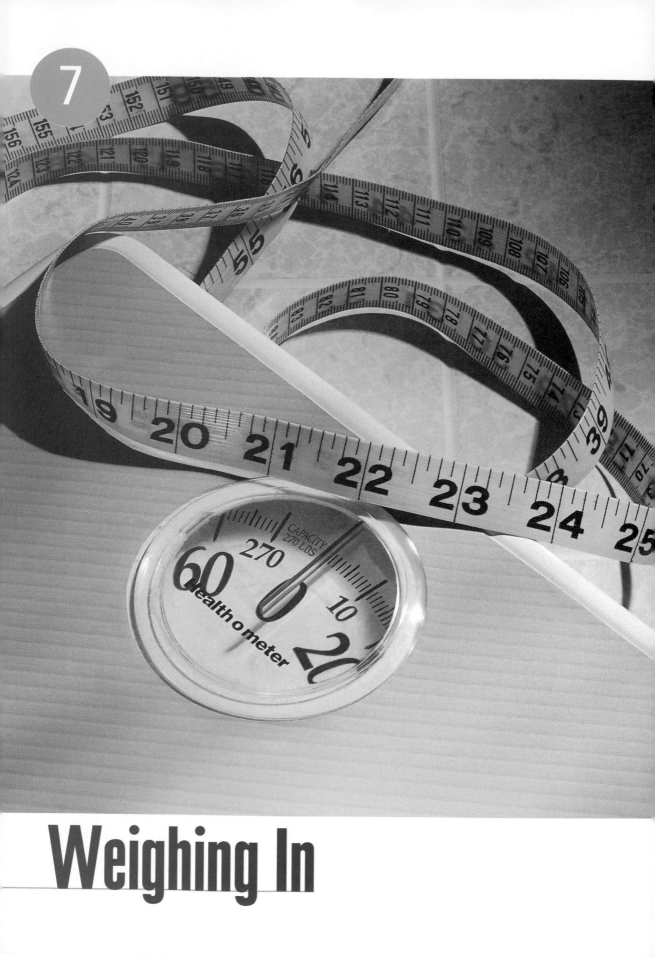

7

Weighing In

Your heart may not be your first reason for wanting to lose weight, but perhaps it should be. Shedding even a few excess pounds can lower your cholesterol and blood pressure and dramatically reduce your risk of type II diabetes—significantly cutting your chances of having a heart attack or stroke. Of course, weight loss will also help you look better, feel better, and have more energy.

If you're hoping to lose a little weight—or even a lot—you're not alone. More than half of all Americans say they're on a diet. And while lightening up isn't easy, it's not impossible. There are thousands of success stories from people who've done it. You can do it, too. Despite what dozens of gimmicky diet books tell you, you won't need any secret formula. Nor will you have to banish a long list of foods from your menu, as too many fad diets require.

If you've begun to adopt some heart-smart eating habits and to add more physical activity to your daily routine, you're already on the road to losing weight. To move forward, you'll need to keep a sharper eye on the calories you consume and concentrate on burning more calories by being more active.

That's right, calories. With all the high-protein, sugar-busting, fat-fighting diet plans out there, it's easy to forget that calories are what matter when you're trying to lose weight.

A calorie is a measure of energy. The calories in food are a measure of the energy they contain—the fuel you need in order to function. (A gram of fat contains 9 calories; proteins and carbohydrates contain 4 calories per gram.) The energy your body burns to maintain all its systems and be active is also measured in calories. And it's plain old calories that determine how much you weigh. Consider these facts:

1. If you consume more calories than you burn, your body will store the excess as fat, and you'll gain weight.

2. If you consume fewer calories than you burn, your body will have to burn fat for energy, and you'll lose weight.

3. If you strike a balance between calories in and calories out, you'll maintain a stable weight.

That's all there is to it: the "secret" of body weight, in three very simple equations.

> With all the high-protein, sugar-busting, fat-fighting diet plans out there, it's easy to forget that calories are what matter when you're trying to lose weight.

Why You?

Chances are you've wondered why you have to struggle with your weight when other people you know can eat all they want and stay slim. Certain factors do make it easier for some people to put on the pounds—and a little harder to take them off. Gaining or losing weight is more than just a matter of willpower, in other words. Five factors may play a role.

1. Genes. Being overweight or obese runs in families. If both of your parents wrestle with weight problems, odds are 7 out of 10 you will, too. If only one of your parents is overweight, your odds drop to 4 in 10. If your parents' weight is normal, you have only a 1 in 10 chance of a weight problem. One way researchers know that genes play a powerful role is by looking at identical twins.

RATE YOUR READINESS

How motivated are you to lose weight? To find out, answer the following questions. Then add up the scores beside the answers you've circled.

How do you feel about the prospect of losing weight?
- Very enthusiastic. 4
- Moderately enthusiastic 3
- Willing. 2
- Discouraged 1

How do you rate your chances of reaching your weight-loss goal?
- Excellent 4
- Very good 3
- Good. 2
- Poor. 1

How important do you think losing weight is for your heart?
- Very important 4
- Important. 3
- Somewhat important 2
- Not very important 1

How would you describe your feeling about restricting the amount of food you eat?
- Very willing 4
- Willing. 3
- Resigned 2
- Reluctant 1

How easy is it for you to stop eating, even if there is still food on your plate?
- Very easy 4
- Easy. 3
- Difficult 2
- Almost impossible 1

How willing are you to give up doing something you like in order to have more time for physical activity?
- Very willing 4
- Willing. 3
- Resigned 2
- Reluctant 1

Studies have shown that twins raised apart are very likely to weigh exactly the same when they grow up, no matter how or where they were raised or who raised them.

But genes aren't destiny. Having overweight parents doesn't mean you'll be fat no matter what you do. It does mean you'll probably have to work a little harder to maintain a healthy weight.

2. Glands. "It's a glandular problem," people often used to say about being overweight. The gland in question is the thyroid, which is located in your neck, just above your voice box. The thyroid controls your metabolism, which affects how many calories you burn while you're at rest. Having an overactive thyroid (hyperthyroidism) means you burn more calories than normal. An underactive thyroid (hypothyroidism) causes you to burn fewer than normal.

Which of these statements do think describes your knowledge about what it takes to lose weight and keep it off?
- I know what it takes 4
- I'm pretty sure I know what it takes . . 3
- I'm confused by conflicting advice and diet plans 2
- I don't know what will work for me . . 1

If your favorite food is in the house, how easy is it for you to resist eating it?
- Easy 4
- A struggle, but I can do it 3
- Difficult 2
- Almost impossible 1

Do you have people close to you who will support you in your weight-loss goal?
- Yes, many 4
- A few 3
- One 2
- No 1

Which of the following statements best describes you?
- If I set my mind to do something, I can do it 4
- I'm pretty good at meeting my goals . 3
- Even when my intentions are good, things seem to get in the way 2
- I get easily discouraged 1

A score of **34–40** means you're ready and willing to begin a weight-loss program.

A score of **25–33** means you're almost ready.

A score of **10–24** suggests you could spend some time and effort mentally preparing yourself before you begin.

If your score falls into one of the last two categories, list your reasons for wanting to lose weight. Then add two more benefits you're likely to get. Write down three of the biggest obstacles you face—and at least one strategy to help you overcome each obstacle. Finally, think about occasions when you've changed something in your life. What helped you succeed? How can you use a similar strategy to lose weight?

Some weight problems do stem from an underactive thyroid—but not many. Fewer than 5 percent of overweight or obese people can really blame this gland. If you think you might fall into that category, talk to your doctor. (Other symptoms of underactive thyroid include lethargy, intolerance to cold temperatures, muscle aches, constipation, and fluid retention.) If blood tests reveal an underactive thyroid, medication can set it right. But don't assume it will be a magic bullet. You'll still have to do what everyone does: Balance calories in and calories out.

3. Metabolism. Some people burn more calories than others, even when they're sleeping or doing nothing at all. There are many reasons for this. Muscle tissue requires more energy to maintain than fat does, so if you're muscular, your resting metabolic rate, or RMR, may be a little higher than someone who has little muscle and a lot of fat. (That's one reason exercises that build muscle help you stay slim.) Some people inherit what researchers have dubbed a "thrifty gene"—an inherited tendency to conserve energy greedily. As a result, they have a lower RMR. Sophisticated tests can measure your RMR. But there's not much point to having such a test done, since the weight-loss prescription is the same: Consume fewer calories and burn more.

4. Fat cells. Fat is stored in special cells that make up adipose, or fatty, tissue. Some people have larger-than-normal fat cells; others have more fat cells than normal. An obese person can have around 260 billion fat cells; a slim person may have only 25 billion. If you've been overweight since childhood, there's a good chance that you may have more fat cells than the average person. That doesn't mean you can't shed some of those pounds, however. No one has ever shown that having too many fat cells makes it harder to lose weight.

5. Personality traits. If you tend to eat when you're feeling sad, lonely, or anxious, you're not alone. Many overweight people say they often eat—and overeat—when they're experiencing emotional distress. Psychological factors like this probably play a role in why some people struggle with

Key Finding

You don't have to lose a lot of weight in order to take the burden off your heart. A 1995 University of Pittsburgh study found that when overweight people lost as little as eight pounds, their blood pressure, LDL cholesterol, and triglycerides all went down. At the same time, their HDL cholesterol levels rose, improving the ratio of good to bad cholesterol—exactly the kind of changes that dramatically lower the risk of a heart attack.

BODY MASS INDEX (BMI)

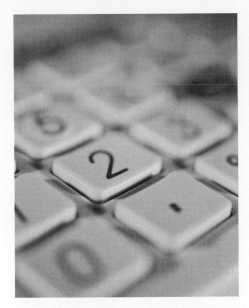

Most people weigh in on the bathroom scale. But those numbers aren't the best measure of healthy weight because they don't take into account height or body type. A more accurate measure is body mass index, or BMI. Follow these instructions to calculate your BMI, or log on to nhlbisupport.com/bmi/bmicalc.htm for a BMI calculator that does the math for you.

1. **Multiply your weight in pounds by 703.**
   Example: 200 x 703 = 140,600
2. **Divide the answer by your height in inches.**
   140,600 ÷ 75 = 1,875
3. **Then divide your answer again by your height in inches.**
   1,875 ÷ 75 = 25

A BMI between 19 and 24 is considered healthy. A BMI between 25 and 29 is considered overweight. A score of 30 or above indicates obesity.

their weight and others don't. By learning to recognize what real hunger feels like (see page 142) and distinguishing it from food cravings, you can go a long way toward eating not to comfort yourself but to satisfy an empty stomach.

Though some or all of these factors may be part of the reason you're overweight, the main culprit is consuming more calories than you burn. Period. If you keep that firmly in mind, you'll have an easier time doing what it takes to lose weight and keep it off.

The Way to Lose Weight

What's the best weight-loss plan for you? Heaven knows there are plenty of them out there, from Dr. Atkins's New Diet Revolution to the Zone. Why so many competing approaches? With more than 100 million frustrated dieters looking for answers, there are big bucks to be made in offering the secret of successful weight loss. Unfortunately, a lot of today's diet plans are based on noth-

PROOF POSITIVE

Diets don't work, the gloomy headlines report. Most people who lose weight gain it back again—and often a few extra pounds as well. Is losing weight a lost cause?

Absolutely not, say James Hill, Ph.D., and Rena Wing, Ph.D., founders of the National Weight Control Registry. Since 1993 they've been inviting people who have successfully lost weight—and kept it off—to share their stories by enrolling in the registry. To qualify, participants must have lost at least 30 pounds and kept it off for at least a year. So far, more than 2,000 people have enrolled. The typical registrant has lost about 60 pounds and kept it off for about 5 years. Most were overweight as children, and 60 percent had a family history of obesity.

Participants fill out a packet of questionnaires, which are then mined for helpful data about what works and what doesn't. "One reason for starting the registry was to counter the prevailing discouraging reports about weight loss with some good news," says Dr. Wing, a professor of psychiatry at Brown University. "Another was to find a way to learn from people who have succeeded about the strategies they used that allowed them to reach and maintain a healthy weight." Here's what the experts are learning:

● Successful weight-losers make significant changes in the way they eat and in their exercise habits.

● Half successfully lose weight on their own without any type of formal program or help.

● On average, people who succeed do so by consuming about 1,400 calories a day and expending about 400 calories a day through physical activity.

● Among weight-losers, walking is the most popular form of exercise.

If you lose at least 30 pounds and keep it off for at least a year, you too can join the registry. Contact the National Weight Control Registry at 1-800-606-NWCR.

ing more than gimmicks. Some of them are downright dangerous, especially if you're at risk for heart disease. For instance, although there is some evidence that high-protein diets do cause people to lose weight at first, protein-rich foods also tend to be loaded with artery-clogging saturated fat.

Look closely at the most popular diet plans, in fact, and you'll discover that nearly all of them offer roughly the same thing: a way to help people cut back on calories. The Zone diet, for instance, contains a long list of foods to avoid, including carrots, corn, peas, sweet potatoes, bananas, raisins, fruit juices, as well as most grains and breads. Ban those foods from your menu and you're almost certain to shed pounds, regardless of the complicated theory behind the diet.

There's a better way to lose weight, however, and it doesn't involve banishing whole categories of foods from your plate. All it takes is making small adjustments to what you eat, how much you eat, and the amount of exercise you get. Over time, those adjustments can add up to a real difference on the scale—and your risk of heart attack. We've put together a four-week program, beginning on page 134, to get you started.

How low should you go?

How much weight can you reasonably expect to lose? If you're overweight or obese, most experts say, it's smart to begin by setting a goal of losing about 10 percent of your current weight. If you weigh 180 pounds, in other words, aim to shed about 18 pounds.

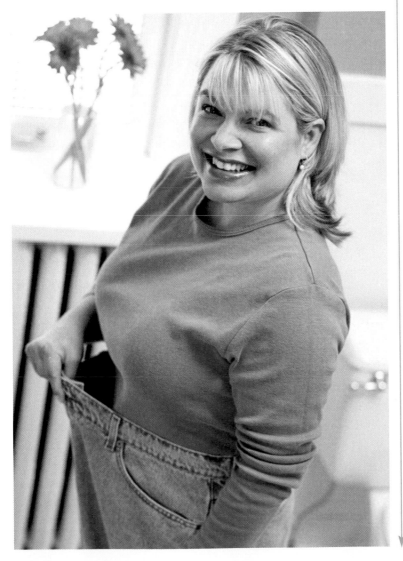

"Most popular diet plans offer roughly the same thing: a way to help people cut back on calories."

If you hit that mark and still have a ways to go to reach your ideal healthy weight, you can always take a deep breath and set another target. Remember: Studies show that losing just 4 percent of body weight can dramatically lower elevated blood pressure and cholesterol levels—which reduces your risk of heart disease and other chronic illnesses.

How fast should you aim to shed those pounds? Researchers say it's both reasonable and safe to lose up to a pound or two a week. To do that, you'll need to consume fewer calories and burn more calories through exercise.

Week One: Keeping a Food and Activity Diary

To shift your calorie balance toward weight loss, it helps to know how many calories you now consume and roughly how many you burn. The Food and Activity Diary on page 137 is designed to help you do that. We recommend making a month's worth of photocopies of the diary and placing them in a looseleaf notebook.

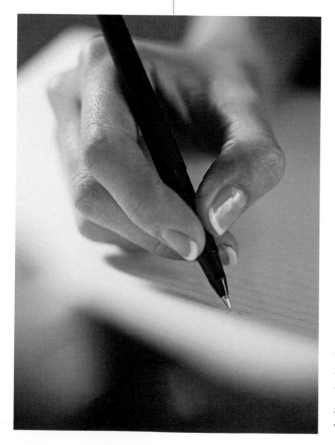

During this first week, concentrate on making note of everything you eat and exactly how much time you spend doing physical activities. Tracking your food intake will help you recognize the food choices you make and the calories they involve. If you find yourself cutting back on portion sizes or skipping that rich dessert because you're suddenly aware of how many calories it contains, fine. But don't start dieting in earnest just yet.

Packaged-food labels state precise calorie counts per serving. But for fresh foods you'll need to buy a calorie counter—a book that lists thousands of foods and the calories they contain. Many bookstores have them. We also recommend buying a small notebook you can carry around to jot down what and how much you eat during the day. Then, at the end of the day fill in your

DIET VS. EXERCISE

To lose weight and keep it off you'll need to exercise and watch your calorie intake. Still, many people find it helps to start by concentrating more on one approach or the other. Each has its advantages. If you're in a hurry to drop pounds, for instance, dieting should be your first plan of attack since it offers quicker results. Plus, it's easier for most people to cut back on the calories they consume than to burn an equivalent number through physical activity. If you're more concerned with how you look in the mirror than with numbers on the scale, exercise may be the way to go, since it tones your muscles while burning fat. Read the following statements and check "Yes" or "No" to determine where to focus your efforts.

❧ I prepare most of my meals at home. Yes ■ No ■

❧ My main goal is to look and feel more toned. Yes ■ No ■

❧ I really want to see those pounds come off, so I plan to measure my progress on the scale. Yes ■ No ■

❧ I'm under a lot of stress, and it sometimes gets me down. Yes ■ No ■

❧ I'm good at planning ahead, especially when it comes to where and what I'll be eating for breakfast, lunch, and dinner. Yes ■ No ■

❧ When I sit down to a meal, I have a tough time saying no to foods I love. Yes ■ No ■

❧ My schedule is hectic, which makes it hard for me to set aside time for myself every day. Yes ■ No ■

❧ I enjoyed sports and other physical activities when I was younger. Yes ■ No ■

❧ I have back problems or other physical conditions that make it hard for me to be very active. Yes ■ No ■

❧ I'm not very good at keeping track of things like calories or fat grams. Yes ■ No ■

❧ I've tried dieting before, and it just hasn't worked for me. Yes ■ No ■

❧ The main reason I want to lose weight is to lower my risk of heart disease. Yes ■ No ■

❧ I've gotten so heavy that I'm embarrassed to be seen even just out walking. Yes ■ No ■

❧ I eat a lot more fast food and junk food than I should. Yes ■ No ■

❧ I'm so out of shape that I just don't have the energy and strength for things that I'd like to do. Yes ■ No ■

Scoring: Add up the number of answers that fall in green boxes and the number in blue boxes. If nine or more of your answers are in green boxes, you're best suited to a program that emphasizes exercise. If nine or more are blue, a program that focuses on diet may work for you. If your answers are more evenly divided between blues and greens, start off with a program that combines diet and exercise.

diary, including the number of calories you've consumed and the number you've expended doing physical activities (see the chart page 122 in Chapter 6 to help you estimate this, or, for a more complete list of activities and how many calories they burn, log onto www.caloriecontrol.org/exercalc.html).

At the end of the week, look back over your diary. You may be surprised at how many calories you expend. Or you may be startled to see how many you consume. The point of this first week is to gauge what your calorie intake and activity level are now. Take a few minutes to calculate the average number of calories you consume each day (add up the seven daily totals and divide by seven). Do the same to calculate the average number of calories you expend through physical activity.

SAMPLE FOOD AND ACTIVITY DIARY

Use the form at right to keep track of the calories you consume and those you expend through exercise. Here's an example of what one day's entries might look like.

TIME OF DAY	FOOD	SERVING SIZE	CALORIES CONSUMED	ACTIVITY	TIME SPENT	CALORIES EXPENDED
6:30 AM	• Orange juice • GrapeNuts • Skim milk • Coffee (black)	½ cup 1 cup ½ cup 8 oz	60 90 43 0			
7:15–7:30				Brisk walk	15 minutes	105
10:00	• Donut	1 small	250			
12:30–1:30 PM	• Tuna sandwich with lettuce and tomato • Diet Pepsi	1 12-oz can	450 0			
3:30	• Apple	1	81			
6:00–6:30				Stationary cycling	30 minutes	300
7:30	• Salmon steak • Pasta with tomato sauce • Green beans • Whole-wheat bread • Wine • Sherbet	3 oz ½ cup ½ cup 2 slices 3 oz ½ cup	120 270 25 80 66 132			
TOTAL			1,667			405

FOOD AND ACTIVITY DIARY

TIME OF DAY	FOOD	SERVING SIZE	CALORIES CONSUMED	ACTIVITY	TIME SPENT	CALORIES EXPENDED

Week Two: Easing Back on Calories

During the second week, your goal is to begin to reduce the calories you consume. Simple, right? Just eat less. That's certainly one strategy. But it's also important to make sure you don't go hungry. Otherwise, you won't last long on your weight-loss plan.

By making savvy food choices, you can sometimes eat more and still come up with fewer calories. For instance, a half cup of Ben & Jerry's Peanut Butter Cup ice cream weighs in at 370 calories. Choose Borden's Strawberries 'N Cream ice milk, which packs only 130 calories in the same serving size, and you can help yourself to a full cup and still rack up

HOT TOPIC

Extreme Dieting

Just as some diet approaches promote high protein consumption, others trumpet the virtues of a very low-fat regimen. There are diets that focus on carbohydrates and diets built around certain foods. Do any of these approaches help people lose weight faster or more easily?

Some foods do seem to satisfy hunger on fewer calories than others. Protein, for instance, has been shown to trigger satiety, or the sense of fullness, faster than fat. And high-fiber foods, like vegetables and whole grains, fill you up faster than foods with little or no fiber.

But there's precious little evidence that diets very high in this or very low in that offer any special benefits when it comes to losing weight and keeping it off. Consider a study conducted

by researchers at Geneva University Hospital in Switzerland. One group of volunteers was given a diet made up of 32 percent protein, 15 percent carbohydrates, and 53 percent fat. The second group ate a diet composed of 29 percent protein, 45 percent carbohydrates, and 26 percent fat. Even on these very different diets—one with only 15 percent and the other with 45 percent of calories from carbohydrates—all volunteers lost the same amount of weight and the same amount of body fat.

What really matters, many experts now say, is how many calories you consume, not where they come from. The best diet for that is one that strikes a reasonable balance—and one you can live with for the rest of your life.

fewer calories. One serving of potato salad at a leading restaurant chain contains 390 calories. Order the steamed vegetables, which contain only 48 calories, and you can have a plateful.

How many calories a day should you aim for? The answer depends partly on how many calories you burn, of course. For women, a weight-loss diet should contain roughly 1,200 calories. For men (because they typically burn more calories), a reasonable goal is about 1,500 calories. According to data from the National Weight Control Registry, people who successfully lose weight and keep it off consume around 1,400 calories a day. Many begin by cutting back to about 1,200, then gradually increasing their intake as they reach their goal.

Look back at your diary to see the average number of calories you consumed each day. If you averaged more than 500 calories over the goal of 1,200 (for women) or 1,500 (for men), you may want to ease yourself down to the new target. For this week, set a goal halfway between what you consumed last week and the target goal. If you're within 500 calories, you're close enough to set 1,200 or 1,500 calories a day as your goal.

Filling up on less

Unless you're eating packaged food, it's not easy to know how many calories an item contains. But you don't always have to. A few simple rules can help guide you toward the foods more likely to fill you up on fewer calories.

1. Reach for foods high in fiber. A bowl of oatmeal is more likely to satisfy your hunger than a bowl of Sugar Pops. A three-bean salad will fill you up faster on fewer calories than a similar-size portion of macaroni salad. That's because foods loaded with fiber satisfy a hearty appetite on fewer calories than low-fiber foods. One reason is that fiber tends to absorb water, so it expands in your stomach. High-fiber foods are also more filling because it takes your stomach longer to break them down into useable energy than almost any other food, so you feel full longer because your stomach is full longer. Some fibers (found in bran, whole grains, vegetables, and the skins of fruits) can't be digested at all. These fibers fill you up without adding any calories to your diet.

139

2. Go easy on fats. Fatty food isn't the only culprit when it comes to body fat. You can put on pounds eating carbohydrates and protein, too. But there's a good reason to go easy on fats, especially saturated fats. A gram of fat packs 9 calories compared to only 4 calories per gram of carbohydrates. Your body also burns about 25 percent more calories digesting carbohydrates than fat. Start by looking for ways to eliminate saturated fats. Enjoy bread without slathering butter on it. Order fish or chicken that's roasted or grilled, not fried. Help yourself to sherbet or ice milk instead of ice cream. To lose weight, you may also need to reduce your intake of heart healthy unsaturated fats as well. Instead of pouring on salad dressing, for instance, drizzle just enough to moisten the leaves and give them added flavor.

3. Favor complex over simple carbohydrates. All carbohydrates are eventually broken down into glucose. But not all carbohydrates are created equal. The simple kind are made up of only one or two sugar molecules. Complex carbohydrates consist of long chains of linked sugars. These take much longer for the body to break down. As a result, blood-sugar levels climb more slowly and remain elevated longer, heading off hunger. Instead of a sugary soft drink, reach for V-8 juice, for instance. And opt for whole-grain instead of white bread.

4. Choose nutrient-dense foods. Especially when you're cutting back on calories, it's important to make sure you get all the nutrition you need. That's why you should choose foods rich in nutrients and not just empty calories. A one-ounce serving of dry-roasted peanuts contains 169 calories—about the same number of calories in a similar-size serving of potato chips. But nuts are loaded with vitamin E, protein, and heart healthy unsaturated fats—unlike chips, which offer little in the way of nutrition. Surprisingly, studies have shown that people who often help themselves to nuts typically weigh less than people who avoid nuts. Even a small handful can be more satisfying than a stack of fat-free crackers.

5. Pump up the volume. Foods that take up a lot of space (think popcorn or a bowl of soup) tend to satisfy hunger on fewer calories, according to Pennsylvania State University nutrition researcher Barbara Rolls, Ph.D., coauthor of *Volumetrics*. In a 2000 study Dr. Rolls found that men who ate yogurt milk shakes whipped up with air in the morning ate less at lunch. The more

> "Surprisingly, studies have shown that people who often help themselves to nuts typically weigh less than people who avoid nuts."

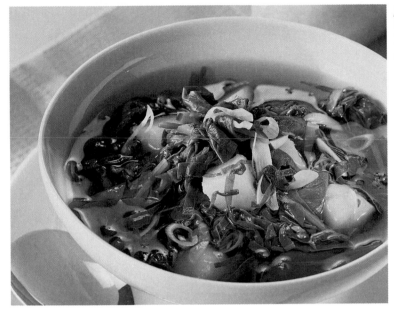

Start dinner off with a bowl of broth-based soup, and you'll consume fewer calories in total by the end of the meal.

Ten High-Volume, Low-Calorie Foods

1. Air-popped popcorn
2. Broth-based soups
3. Cream-of-wheat cereal
4. Most fruits (except dried fruits)
5. Green vegetables
6. Low-fat yogurt
7. Puffed-wheat cereal
8. Unsweetened tea
9. Tomatoes
10. Vegetable juice

air the shakes contained (and thus the more volume they had), the fuller the men felt afterward. Dr. Rolls has also shown that people feel full longer after having a bowl of chicken and rice soup than they do after eating a chicken and rice casserole with exactly the same number of calories. The reason: Broth is mostly water, so it fills you up on very few calories.

Join the slow food movement

Not long ago, food lovers from around the world founded a new movement called Slow Food. Its aim: to counter the trend toward fast-food eating habits. The Slow Food movement encourages people to cherish the joys of good food by finding better tasting (and healthier) alternatives to, say, burgers and fries—and taking the time to savor every mouthful.

Think about your eating habits. Chances are you've often grabbed something to eat and bolted it down without ever paying attention to how it tastes. All those calories—and you never even took a moment to enjoy them! This week, try to slow down and pay attention whenever you sit down to eat. Follow these few simple tips, and you're likely to consume less and enjoy it a lot more.

Drop everything else. When it's time to eat, eat. Don't have a meal while you're watching TV. Or eat while you're driving. Or do a crossword puzzle while gobbling down lunch. Sit down somewhere and give the meal or snack all your attention. People who

141

eat while distracted by other activities typically overeat because they're not paying enough attention to know when they've had enough to be satisfied—not stuffed.

Stick to a schedule. Whenever possible, have your meals at roughly the same hour every day. Some people find it even helps to schedule meals, the way they schedule meetings. By setting aside a particular time to eat, you'll give the meal the priority it deserves.

Put your fork down between bites. Eat too quickly, and you won't give your body the chance to register the calories you've consumed and to send your brain the message that you've had enough. In fact, one big reason many of us eat too much, experts say, is that we eat too fast. Remember: It can take up to 20 minutes for your body to signal that you're full. Putting your silverware down between bites will help keep you in the slow lane.

Serve smaller portions. At home, cut your standard portion sizes in half (you can go back for more if you're still hungry). After you've finished the first serving, take five minutes to relax before getting up for more. Before you do, think about whether you're really hungry. Help yourself if you are. If not, leave the table.

If it doesn't taste wonderful, don't eat it. When you're cutting back on calories, every bite counts. If you don't love what you're eating, put it aside.

Never feel you have to clean your plate. Instead of beginning a meal with the goal of finishing what's in front of you, begin with the goal of satisfying your hunger. As soon as you no longer feel hungry, put down your fork and get up from the table.

Eat only when you're hungry

When energy stores dip low, the body sends out physical signals in the form of hunger pangs to remind us to take in calories. Unfortunately, most of us rarely wait that long. We help ourselves to food not because we're physically hungry but because of all

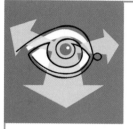

LOOKING AHEAD

A prickly weight-loss solution

For thousands of years the Hoodia cactus, a native plant of South Africa, has been used by bushmen to stave off hunger during long hunting trips. Someday it could provide a boon to Westerners seeking to lose weight. Scientists have isolated one of the plant's active chemical compounds, dubbed P57, thought to suppress appetite. The compound is now in the early stages of testing in humans.

FIVE FLAVORFUL WAYS
TO CUT CALORIES

Low-fat foods don't have to be bland. Talented chefs use several tricks to give food big flavor without adding unnecessary fat or calories. You can, too. Here's how.

■ **Choose high-flavor ingredients.** An aged reggiano cheese costs a little more than parmesan in the shaker can, but it also delivers a bigger flavor bang, so you'll need less to make a dish satisfying. Smoked mozzarella has twice the taste of the plain kind, so a little bit goes a long way on homemade pizza. Instead of adding hamburger meat to spaghetti sauce, buy a highly seasoned hard Italian sausage and dice a few pieces for a flavorful meal with less fat. Use reconstituted dried mushrooms in savory dishes for a concentrated taste sensation. Add a splash of sherry or wine to sauces to boost flavor without adding fat.

■ **Splurge on herbs.** Rich doesn't have to mean buttery. Experiment with herbs and seasonings to entertain your taste buds. A simple lentil and vegetable soup simmered with fresh oregano, thyme, and a bay leaf makes a hearty meal. Dried currants or raisins and a smattering of Middle Eastern spices like cumin or cardamom turn rice into an exotic dish. Rosemary brings delicious accent to chicken dishes, potatoes, and roasted vegetables. If fresh herbs are hard to find or too expensive, used dried herbs, or consider starting a window-box herb garden with a few of your favorites.

■ **Chop it up.** By slicing and dicing ingredients into small pieces, you'll release more of their flavor and increase the volume of the dish, making a medium-size portion seem bigger. (Another trick to make a modest meal seem opulent: Serve it on smaller plates.)

■ **Less is more.** In traditional Mediterranean and Asian cultures, meat was hard to come by, so home cooks learned simple ways to make a little go a long way. Try combining a small amount of diced hard sausage with beans in a pasta sauce or tossing in plenty of vegetables and tofu along with a bit of chicken for an easy stir fry.

■ **Be colorful.** What chefs love best about fruits and vegetables are the colors they bring to a meal. Nutritionists celebrate them because they're low in calories and fat and high in fiber, which makes a meal feel more filling. You can brighten up almost any dish— from tuna casserole to a breakfast omelet—by adding chopped broccoli, corn, asparagus, or diced tomatoes.

kinds of psychological cues. If you're used to having a tub of pop-corn every time you go to the movies, for instance, you'll crave one as soon as you buy your ticket—even if you've just had dinner.

"A lot of the people we see in our weight-loss programs have never really learned to identify true hunger," says John Foreyt, Ph.D., a weight-loss expert at Baylor College of Medicine in Houston, Texas. "They misconstrue all kinds of other feelings as hunger—which means they often eat even when they aren't really

A LOW-CAL MENU THAT WON'T STARVE YOU

How well can you eat and still stay under 1,400 calories a day? Let's face it, you won't be snacking on Krispy-Kreme donuts or indulging in a chocolate decadence for dessert. But you can enjoy three satisfying meals—with a couple of healthy snacks thrown in. Here's what a typical under-1,400-calorie menu looks like.

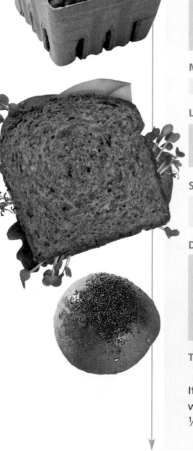

FOOD	SERVING SIZE	CALORIES
BREAKFAST		
All Bran with extra fiber	1 cup	100
Skim milk	½ cup	42
Blueberries	¼ cup	20
Orange juice	6 oz	50
MIDMORNING SNACK		
Apple or pear	1 medium	81
LUNCH		
Turkey sandwich on whole-wheat bread with lettuce and tomato		275
Diet cola	12 oz	0
SNACK		
V-8 juice	6 oz	35
Roasted cashews	1 oz	150
DINNER		
Turkey meat loaf	1 slice	196
Leafy green salad with 2 Tbsp vinaigrette		100
Green beans and carrots lightly sautéed in ½ Tbsp olive oil	1 cup	100
Whole-wheat dinner roll	1 small	100
Sherbet	1 cup	150
TOTAL:		1359

If your goal is 1,200 calories a day, replace the roasted cashews with 2 cups of air-popped popcorn (about 35 calories) and have a ½ cup of frozen grapes (35 calories) instead of sherbet.

physically hungry." According to Dr. Foreyt, we often eat when we're feeling stressed, or lonely, or bored, or anxious.

Can you resist all those psychological cues and eat only when you're hungry? Absolutely, the experts say. But first it helps to know what real hunger feels like—and the simplest way to do that is to skip a meal. When you're truly hungry, your stomach feels empty. Chances are you'll begin to feel distracted, preoccupied with the thought of eating.

What about those times you find yourself ravenous for chocolate or something salty? No, you're not genuinely hungry; you're experiencing a psychological craving. When that happens, change what you're doing or where you are. Get up and take a quick walk or do a couple of chores around the house. Often the craving will pass. Then you can wait until your body needs food before you raid the refrigerator.

Reaching your calories goal

At the end of week two, look back over your daily calorie consumption. If you met your goal, congratulations. If not, don't be discouraged. You're making progress simply by becoming aware of what you eat and how many calories your meals contain. If you still have a ways to go to bring your calorie consumption down:

- Review your food diary and identify at least three items you can live without. Eliminate foods low in nutrients and high in calories, like sweets or salty snacks.
- Identify at least three items you can eat less of by cutting back on portion size.
- Identify at least one food that can be replaced with something lower in calories. If your breakfast cereal contains more than 200 calories per serving, for instance, try a puffed wheat or a rice cereal, which fills a bowl with under 100 calories.
- Plan to eat at least one additional serving of vegetables a day this coming week, either steamed or very lightly sautéed in olive or canola oil. The fiber in vegetables will help fill you up on the fewest possible calories, so you'll be less tempted by higher-fat, higher-calorie foods.

Week Three: Burning More Calories

You're on your way to controlling the calories you consume. Now it's time to turn your attention to the other side of the calorie balance equation: the calories you burn. Most studies show that the only reliable way to lose weight and keep it off is to diet and exercise. Why? By burning additional calories through physical activity, you can increase the number of calories you consume and still maintain a healthy weight. The result: being able to enjoy a satisfying amount of food.

Any physical activity will do. The exercise of choice among most of the people enrolled in the National Weight Control Registry is walking. On average, successful weight-losers burn about 400 calories a day through exercise. For a 150-pound person, that means walking four to five miles at a brisk pace—roughly an hour's worth of walking—every day.

Look back at your Food and Activity Diary for last week. Tabulate the calories you burned each day. Then calculate an average by adding the daily totals and dividing by 7. Subtract that number from 400 to see how many additional calories you need to burn in order to reach the goal of 400 a day.

This week, seek any opportunity, however brief, to expend calories. Take the stairs instead of the escalator. Even doing jumping jacks or jogging in place for four minutes instead of sitting on the couch during the TV commercials will help. Of course, the more vigorous the activity—and the longer you engage in it—the more calories you burn. Use your Food and Activity Diary to keep track of calories in and calories out.

TROUBLESHOOTING TIP

Not shedding pounds as fast as you'd like? Don't get discouraged. For some people, losing weight takes more time than for others. Even if the numbers on the scale haven't budged, as long as you're adding more exercise to your life, you're losing fat and replacing it with muscle. And that will make it easier to keep the pounds off once you do begin losing weight.

Week Four: Staying on Track

Look over your diary for the past week and add up your calorie tallies (both calories consumed and calories expended) to see how close you came to meeting your goal. If you didn't quite hit the numbers you were hoping for, identify some of the obstacles that hindered you. Then brainstorm a few strategies to get around them. For example:

WAYS TO BURN 400 CALORIES

A surefire way to burn 400 calories is by taking a long, brisk walk. Turn this into a daily habit and your work is done. On the other hand, you don't have to expend those calories all at once. Here are some different scenarios, based on a 150-pound person.

ACTIVITY	TIME		CALORIES
Brisk walking	65 minutes		400
		TOTAL	400
Brisk walking	30 minutes		180
Sweeping sidewalk	10 minutes		50
Bowling	45 minutes		150
Vacuuming	5 minutes		20
		TOTAL	400
Brisk walking	30 minutes		180
Low-impact aerobic dance	30 minutes		180
Climbing stairs	5 minutes		40
		TOTAL	400
Vacuuming	15 minutes		60
Raking leaves	10 minutes		100
Swimming easy laps	30 minutes		240
		TOTAL	400

Can't find the time for exercise? Think of ways to turn downtime into active time. Arrange to meet friends for a walk instead of talking on the phone. Buy a stationary bike so you can pedal while watching your favorite TV show.

Having trouble keeping track of what you eat? Buy a small notebook that you can fit into your pocket and bring it everywhere you go.

Are restaurant meals your downfall? Identify a few local restaurants that offer delicious low-calorie choices and reward them with your business.

Overwhelmed by trying to change so many things? You're not alone. Most people have trouble tackling too many lifestyle changes at once. It helps to start with just one change; once you have that one down, you can move on to another.

Remember: Everyone has good days and bad days—periods when they stick to their goals and periods when they struggle. But people who succeed over the long term have one thing in common: They remain firmly committed to their goal even in the face of occasional setbacks. The more determined you are to lose weight, the more likely you are to succeed.

FAST FACT

When people diet without exercising, they lose not only fat but also muscle—which in turn slows down their metabolism, causing them to burn fewer calories.

147

Adjusting your goals

Over the coming weeks and months, continue to keep track of the calories you consume and expend. Along the way, you may find yourself losing weight steadily and then suddenly hitting a plateau, where the pounds don't come off as easily or where your weight

REAL PEOPLE, REAL WISDOM

Secrets of a Successful Loser

"I've always been a little chunky," says Karen Langlais, 52. "But after I turned 30, I began to gain weight. I'd quit smoking. My metabolism was slowing down. The combination meant I was putting on about 6 pounds a year. By the time I hit 40, I was 200 pounds. I looked at myself in the mirror one day and said, 'No way I'm going to be fat at 50.' "

It wasn't just the way she looked that worried her. She'd quit smoking to protect her heart and lungs; she didn't want to risk a heart attack now because of all the weight she'd gained. Lately, too, she'd noticed that she was getting much more winded when she and her husband went hiking together.

As it happened, Langlais had been hounding her sister to quit smoking. So the two of them struck a deal. If Langlais could get down to her ideal weight of 120, her sister would give up cigarettes.

Just about that time, Langlais heard about a weight-loss study being conducted by the University of Pennsylvania. Figuring she could use all the help she could get, she enrolled. She was instructed to keep her daily calorie intake at around 1,000 calories. She was also told to begin walking 10 miles each week and gradually increase that distance to 25 miles a week.

By the end of the first month, she'd lost 10 pounds. Within eight months she'd reached her goal of 120 pounds. Once there, she switched to a maintenance diet of 1,800 calories a day—1,400 in the winter, when she finds that it's harder to get exercise. Two years after starting the program, she's still at her target weight. Her resting heart rate, which had climbed to almost 90 beats a minute, is now a much healthier 67. Her blood pressure has also fallen a few points.

What's the secret of her success? "One thing you have to do is keep track. After the first year, I decided to stop counting calories—and right away I began to gain weight again," says Langlais. Another secret: learning to design her menu around the produce aisle. "I know it sounds silly, but I've really learned to love fruits and vegetables and all the ways you can fix them. I've actually come to enjoy eating even more than I used to, because now I pay attention and enjoy everything I eat."

Langlais's success yielded one more important benefit: Her sister stopped smoking.

remains stuck where it is. Don't be discouraged. Almost everyone who has a significant amount of weight to lose hits a plateau.

The best advice, say experts, is to relax for a bit, celebrate the progress you've made, and stick to your calorie goals. After a little while, you may see the pounds coming off again. If not, increase the calories you burn by adding 15 minutes of exercise a day. A brisk 15-minute walk will help you burn an extra 75 to 100 calories. Or cut 100 calories from your diet by adjusting a portion size or eliminating a snack.

Once you reach your weight goal, you can adjust your diet again, this time gradually increasing the number of calories you consume. Why? Because in order to lose weight, you must consume fewer calories than you actually need so

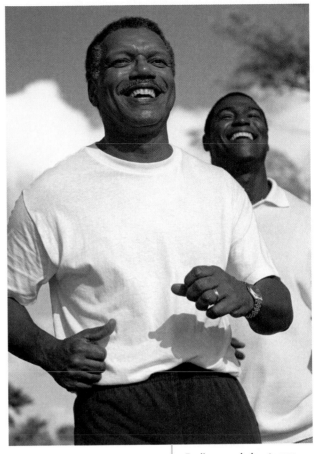

Feeling good about your new habits? Great! If you think of yourself as an active person who cares about eating well, you can use that new self-image to help you stay the course.

that you'll force your body to burn fat for energy. To maintain your new weight, you need only to strike a balance between the calories you consume and those you burn. That usually means being able to boost your calorie intake just a tad. How much depends on your ideal weight and how active you are. If you're a woman, try setting your maintenance level at 1,800 calories a day. If you're a man, set a goal of 2,100 calories a day. If you notice yourself beginning to gain weight, you'll need to increase your activity level or lower your calorie intake.

Don't be surprised if you find yourself having to adjust your diet or your activity level now and then. Most people who have successfully lost weight, especially those who have shed a significant number of pounds, say they have to continue to keep an eye on the calories they consume and push themselves to stay active. (That's why it's important that you really enjoy the form of exercise you choose—it's a long-term proposition!) And don't be alarmed if you put on a few pounds during life's rough spots. You've lost the weight before, and you can do it again.

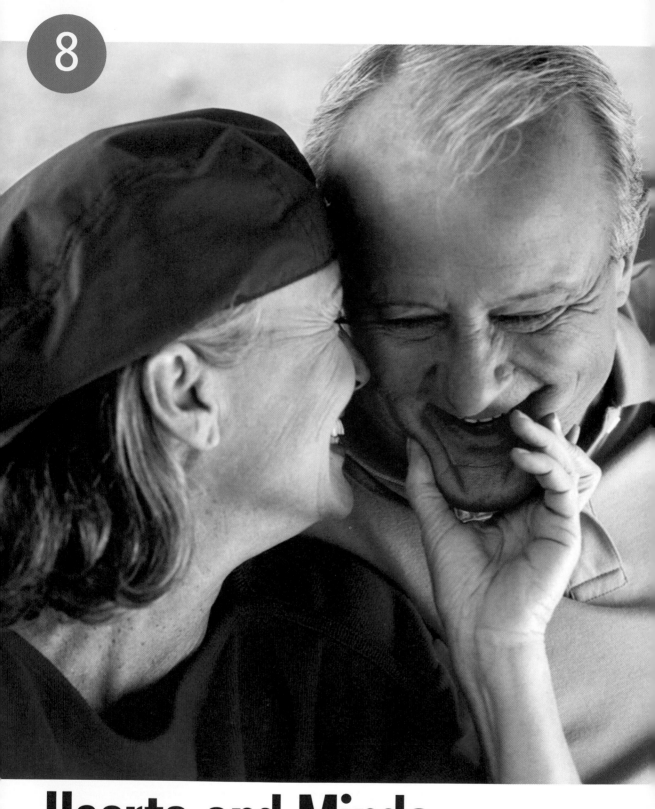

8

Hearts and Minds

The heart has long been linked with our emotions. When we're feeling sad, we say we're downhearted. When our feelings are there for everyone to see, we're wearing our heart on our sleeve. Now medical researchers have begun turning up powerful connections between our state of mind and the health of our heart. How is your outlook affecting yours?

Dozens of studies have shown that negative emotions such as anger or depression increase heart disease danger. People suffering from depression may be as much as four times more likely than others to have a heart attack. Heart attacks also occur much more frequently in people coping with a divorce or separation. Anger and anxiety, too, seem to put a strain on the heart.

But if negative emotions threaten the heart, positive ones seem to protect it. People who are able to laugh at situations they encounter are at less risk of heart disease than sourpusses who rarely chuckle, according to findings published in 2001 in the *International Journal of Cardiology*. In another study, researchers looking at a group of almost 600 people with a family history of heart disease found that those who were optimistic were half as likely as their grumpier counterparts to develop heart problems.

> People who are able to laugh at situations they encounter are at less risk of heart disease than sourpusses who rarely chuckle.

Stress: Hard on Your Heart

What forges the link between hearts and minds? Researchers don't have all the answers, but many believe that part of the connection is a physical reaction known as the stress response. When we're afraid or feeling threatened, our bodies go into high gear to prepare us for action. Our hearts begin to pound. Blood pressure increases. A hormone called adrenaline, which is a powerful stimulant, surges into the bloodstream. At the same time, glucose, fat, and cholesterol are released into the blood in case we need extra energy. Chemical changes in the blood make it more likely to clot, possibly to stanch bleeding in the event of injury.

All these events are part of what psychologists call the fight-or-flight response. In the early days of human evolution, fighting or fleeing were usually the only choices we had in the face of danger. Even today, in situations of real physical peril, like a fire or a

Signs of Stress

1. Fatigue
2. Frequent headaches
3. Sleeplessness
4. Loss of appetite
5. Loss of sense of humor
6. Irritability or anger
7. Fidgeting or pacing
8. Increased eating or smoking
9. Blaming others
10. Shouting or swearing
11. Throwing things
12. Shakiness in your hands
13. Trouble

speeding car, the fight-or-flight response can be lifesaving. But more often than not, the hazards we perceive are psychological. We worry about our jobs, our families, or our health. These stresses can set off the same bodily reactions as those triggered by a physical threat. And if we live in a constant state of worry or anxiety, researchers speculate, the stress response can harm the heart. A racing heartbeat and elevated blood pressure may cause turbulence in the bloodstream that can damage artery walls, making them more vulnerable to the buildup of plaque, for example. The rush of glucose and cholesterol into the bloodstream may compound the problem.

It's well known that both physical and emotional stress can trigger angina or even a heart attack in people with serious coronary artery disease. Here's how: The combination of a pounding heartbeat and rising blood pressure increases the heart's need for oxygen. If coronary arteries are narrowed, they may not be able to supply the extra blood, and this can result in chest pain. Stress also triggers the release of fibrin, a substance that makes blood clot more easily, and this could contribute to the formation of a clot in the coronary artery, causing a heart attack. Many people with coronary artery disease experience both angina and heart attacks during or immediately following periods of stress.

To test the link between anxiety and heart attacks, researchers at the University of California at San Diego conducted a clever experiment. They tallied up the number of deaths that occurred on the fourth day of each month, between 1973 and 1998. Why the fourth? Because many Chinese and Japanese consider the number 4 unlucky. (In Mandarin,

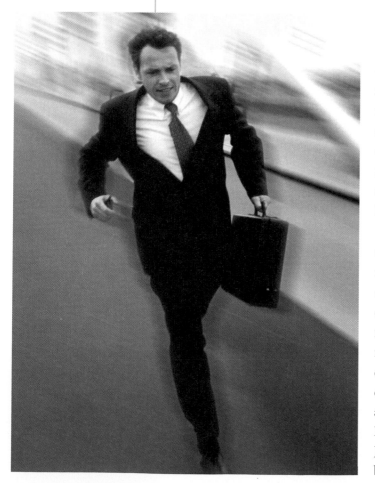

ARE YOU A HOTHEAD?

Is the way you react to stress putting your heart at risk? Imagine yourself in the following situations. Even though they may not apply to your life, think about whether you might be likely to respond in the manner described.

❧ The appliance company promises to deliver your new dishwasher between 10:00 A.M. and noon, and now it's 2:00 P.M. You've called twice and left a message, and no one has called back. You can feel your heart racing and your stomach churning with anger.

Yes ■ No ■

❧ You've agreed to meet two friends for dinner before a concert, and they're already 15 minutes late. If they don't come soon, you may not have time to eat and get to the performance. You become so frustrated and annoyed that when they finally arrive you can't relax enough to enjoy dinner.

Yes ■ No ■

❧ You're trying to get something done at your desk, and your spouse keeps coming into the room and interrupting you. Finally you've had enough, and you angrily demand to be left alone.

Yes ■ No ■

❧ Your boss came down hard on you for not being prepared. You are so angry afterward that your hands are trembling, and you can feel yourself perspiring. You even find yourself thinking of ways to get back at your boss.

Yes ■ No ■

❧ Just when you need a little support and encouragement, your spouse treats you coldly. Instead of saying something directly, you silently fume about the way you've

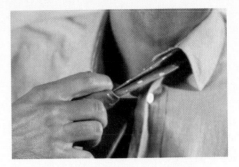

been treated, feeling more and more resentful.

Yes ■ No ■

❧ Two friends you've invited to dinner call at the last minute to cancel, saying they're under the weather. The meal is almost prepared, the table is set. You can practically feel your blood pressure climb. You vow never to see these friends again.

Yes ■ No ■

❧ At a movie theater, the couple in front of you keeps talking loud enough to disturb you. You could move to another seat. But their rudeness is so infuriating to you that you lean forward and angrily tell them to shut up.

Yes ■ No ■

❧ You're in the middle of a phone conversation when your friend puts you on hold to get another call. Thirty seconds pass, then a minute, and you can feel your irritation mounting. Finally you've had enough, and you slam the phone down.

Yes ■ No ■

Scoring: If you answered Yes to five or more of the statements, you may be what psychologists call a hot responder. Instead of remaining patient and calm, you react angrily, your heart rate accelerating and your muscles tensing. The more Yes responses you circled, the more important it is for you to find ways to relax.

Cantonese, and Japanese, the word "four" sounds almost exactly like the word "death.") Sure enough, deaths from heart disease peaked on that day—but only among Chinese and Japanese people, not non-Asian Americans. For people of Chinese or Japanese ancestry who were in the hospital, the death rate was almost 50 percent higher on the fourth of the month than other days. Even fears that most of us would think of as superstitious, it turns out, can even increase heart attack risk.

Is your personality putting you at risk?

All of us experience stress, of course. Bad things happen, to paraphrase a popular bumper sticker. Not everyone develops heart disease as a result. Why do some people seem especially vulnerable? Again, scientists don't have all the answers. But certain personality traits appear to increase the risk. The classic heart disease-prone personality is the Type A. Type A individuals aren't just ambitious, they're driven to succeed. And because they don't want anything to get in their way, they can be aggressive, even hostile. Type As are impatient, easily irritated, and quick to anger. Always in a hurry, they often try to do more than one thing at a time. They talk on the phone while driving, for instance, or read reports while eating.

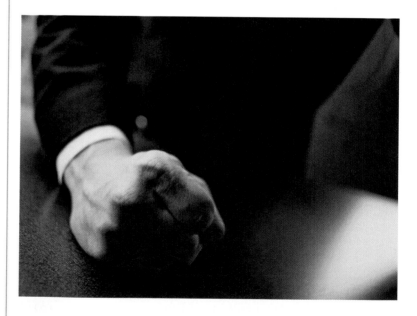

By pushing themselves and others so hard, some research suggests, Type As put a potentially deadly strain on their heart. In a study of 1,305 men, those who scored highest on a test used to measure Type A traits were three times more likely to have a heart

FAST FACT

The most commonly reported incident preceding a heart attack is an emotionally upsetting experience—particularly one involving anger.

attack over the seven years that followed than men who scored at the bottom end of the scale. Although most studies of Type A behavior have involved men, several investigations have looked at Type A women and found similar results.

By the 1980s, Type A behavior was officially listed as an independent risk factor for heart disease, right up there with elevated blood pressure and high levels of bad cholesterol.

Hotheads, take heed

But now many researchers aren't so sure that Type A behavior itself is the real problem. The true threat may be just one aspect of a Type A personality: hostility, or the tendency to react with anger, even at the slightest provocation. An anger-prone person is someone who gets right on the tail of a slow-moving car, honking the horn and even cursing. Or someone who lashes out angrily when a colleague arrives late for an important meeting due to an unavoidable delay.

In a study of 12,986 men and women, researchers found that people who scored high on a standard test to measure anger were more than twice as likely as those who scored low to develop coronary artery disease. In fact, over time chronic anger may pose almost as much risk as smoking. Redford B. Williams, a cardiologist at Duke University Medical School, discovered that physicians who scored in the top half on a hostility questionnaire administered at the age of 25 were four to five times more likely to have heart disease than low scorers by the time they reached age 50.

Why is anger hard on your heart? One possible reason is that being constantly angry is stressful, increasing heart rate and blood pressure. But there may be other reasons. Ohio State University researchers recently found that men and women with high levels of hostility also had higher than normal levels of homocysteine, the blood chemical that is strongly associated with coronary artery

Key Finding

Cooling your head just might save your life, according to findings from the Recurrent Coronary Prevention Program in San Francisco. In that study, heart attack patients prone to Type A behavior were assigned either to a group that received standard counseling on diet and exercise or to a group that received the same counseling along with an intensive stress-management program. Those in the second group were taught how to relax physically and mentally when they felt stress building. They also used role-playing to practice coping skills. Four and a half years later, the people in the stress-management group had suffered half as many heart attacks as those in the control group.

REAL PEOPLE, REAL WISDOM

Prayer for Peace of Mind

Sure, her blood pressure was too high, and her cholesterol levels were in the danger zone. But Josephine Richau is convinced the real reason she has heart disease is too much stress.

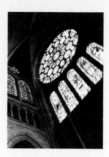

"I've always been a worrier," says Richau, a special-education expert in San Francisco. In recent years she's had plenty of family problems to worry over. When things went wrong for one of her daughters a few years ago, Richau and her husband found themselves raising one of their grandchildren—just about when they'd planned to retire.

"Believe me, it hasn't been easy," says Richau. "There are times when I've been under so much stress and pressure that I slip into a depression and have trouble getting out. Sometimes I can almost feel all the worry putting a strain on my heart."

One day, rushing home to meet her husband, she started to feel a pain in her chest. It gradually subsided when she sat down and rested. But the next day, after experiencing another bout of crushing pain in her chest, she went to the hospital, where she was diagnosed with angina.

"The doctors gave me nitroglycerin pills to take. And for a little while I thought everything was back to normal," says Richau. "But whenever I was under stress, I would experience more angina." In the midst of giving a party for her grandson, she had another bout of chest pain, this time more severe than before. Back at the hospital, Richau underwent an angiogram (an X-ray test that uses dye to create detailed images of the coronary arteries), which showed a severe blockage in one artery.

Today, thanks to an angioplasty—a procedure used to open up blocked arteries—she's feeling 100 percent better. To stay that way, Richau tries to follow a healthy diet that includes more fruits and vegetables and to be as physically active as she can be. She's also making an effort to keep her weight down. "But the most important thing I can do for my heart," she says, "is not become overwhelmed by stress, the way I used to."

Richau admits that's not easy. There are still days when the pressure of family problems leaves her feeling frazzled, and occasions when she gets depressed. "But now, when things get bad, I try to slow down, take a deep breath, and put things in perspective. If it's something I can change, I try to change it. If not, I try to let it go."

The most powerful antidote to stress, for Richau, is prayer. "Some people use a mantra. Some people meditate. I pray. I'm not overly religious, but I have a strong faith. I have a prayer that I say over and over when things get too pressured," she says. "It helps me put all the worry aside and find strength when I'm feeling overwhelmed."

disease. And in a University of Pittsburgh study published in 2001, researchers found that women who scored high on tests that measure anger had a fourfold or greater risk for high LDL and low HDL levels—both strong risk factors for heart disease. Anger has also been shown to make the blood more likely to clot.

The dangers of depression

Like stress, anxiety, and anger, depression can also take a toll on the heart. People who are depressed or socially isolated run up to four times the normal risk of developing coronary artery disease. And once heart disease has set in, people who feel chronically down-in-the-mouth appear more likely to have a heart attack or die of their disease. Consider the results of a Swedish study that followed 275 men and women who had already had one heart attack. Those who scored high on tests that measure depression were three times more likely than their more buoyant counterparts to die of heart disease within a 10-year period.

No one knows exactly how sadness and despair wreak their havoc on the heart. One guess is that depression itself is stressful. Another is that depressed people may be less likely to take care of themselves. University of Pittsburgh researchers recently found that they are almost three times more likely than average to be smokers, for instance. A Johns Hopkins study reported in 2001 showed that heart attack sufferers who are depressed and pessimistic about their health are less likely than cheerier souls to make the diet and lifestyle changes that might protect their hearts.

Symptoms of depression include persistent sadness, loss of interest in pleasurable activities, low energy, insomnia (especially early waking), weight loss or gain, difficulty concentrating, and loss of hope. If you think you might be depressed, talk to your doctor. Psychotherapy and antidepressant medications can help.

Key Finding

Stress tends to raise your heart rate and constrict your blood vessels, contributing to high blood pressure. Slow, deep breathing can reverse this chain of events. Now there's a device that helps you practice it. RespeRate analyzes your breathing through a sensor worn around the midsection, then plays musical tones to guide you through 15-minute breathing exercises that lower your breathing rate. Clinical trials have supported the use of the device, which has been approved by the FDA as an adjunctive treatment for hypertension. It is available only with a prescription from your doctor.

Guarding Your Heart

Not every worrier or hothead is doomed to develop heart disease. And not everyone who lives a stressful life feels overwhelmed. But if your emotions are getting the best of you, it's time to take action.

You can't change who you are, of course. But you can change the way you react to events and situations. The first step is recognizing when stress is becoming a problem. And no one knows that better than you. If you're having trouble sleeping, if the simple pleasures of life don't give you much enjoyment anymore, if you're tired much of the time, you may be suffering from chronic stress. (To rule out other health problems, mention your symptoms to your doctor.)

Next, identify the sources of the worst pressure and strain in your life. (If you feel anxious without really knowing why, and your feelings are so intense that they interfere with your daily functioning, you could be suffering from a condition known as generalized anxiety disorder, which can be treated with medication and/or psychotherapy.) Then take some time to figure out which ones you can eliminate or disarm.

> Sit down with your calendar and find a way to rid yourself of activities you can live without.

Facing stress head-on

If you're worried about money, take a hard look at ways to reorganize your finances or economize. If you and your spouse are going through a rocky time, decide what steps you can take to alleviate the tension—then take them. You may find that making even one move toward alleviating the source of your stress can help restore a sense of control over your situation and even galvanize you to make another one.

Around the house, a little bit of disorganization can cause a lot of aggravation if you can't find something when you need it. Launch preemptive strikes by setting up a filing system for your bills, paperwork, and letters, for instance. Even something as simple as

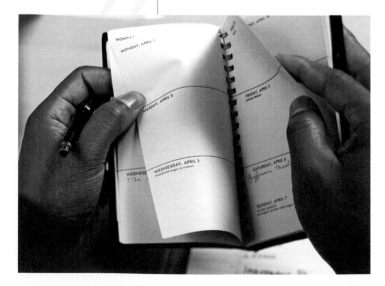

deciding, once and for all, where to keep the car and house keys—and making sure they go there—can make life a little less stressful.

If a crowded schedule or too many commitments is a problem, take charge of your time. Sit down with your calendar and find a way to rid yourself of activities you can live without or delegate responsibilities that could be done by someone else.

Coping for the best

Of course, sometimes it's impossible to weed out the root causes of your stress. That's why it's also important to develop some coping skills. Remember, it's not a stressful situation that harms your health, it's your reaction to it. Here's how to get started.

1. Slow down. The original term for Type A behavior was "hurry syndrome," because hard-driven people tend to do everything faster than more relaxed types. Encourage yourself to relax by consciously slowing your walking pace, driving more slowly, and taking more time to enjoy your meals. The next time you find yourself rushing around, stop, take a deep breath, and slow down.

2. Ease up on yourself. Sometimes we put stress on ourselves by thinking in terms of absolutes, using words like "never" or

SMOOTH MOVES

Feeling stressed out? A yoga class could be the solution. Exercise scientists have long known that yoga offers a great way to stretch your muscles and improve your balance. Now psychologists are showing that it also eases a troubled mind. When researchers from the University of Würzburg in Germany tested 12 women before, during, and after a 60-minute yoga class, they found that the women's heart rates dropped dramatically during the class. The women also reported feeling less irritable.

In fact, yoga may be one of the best ways to improve your sense of well-being. At Oxford University, a psychologist divided 71 men and women into three groups. One group practiced simple relaxation techniques. The second used visualization to imagine themselves feeling less tense. The third did a half-hour yoga routine. The folks in the first two groups reported feeling sluggish afterward. The people in the yoga group, on the other hand, said they felt more energetic and emotionally content.

"should" or "always." I should never have done that, we tell ourselves. She's always late whenever we need to be somewhere. If you notice yourself thinking in absolutes, lighten up. Replace irrational thoughts with more reasonable ones. Things don't always go wrong for you, after all. The truth is, things occasionally go wrong for everyone. And when they do, everyone has the same challenge: to sort things out and get on with life.

3. Let it go. Next time something gets you stressed or angry, take a step back and ask yourself if it's really worth getting worked up about. If it isn't, let it go. If you're a hothead, and you find your

HOT TOPIC

The Healing Power of Forgiveness

Most of us have been hurt by someone in our lives, and many of us have trouble letting go of that hurt. A cruel remark, a deliberately hurtful act, even physical violence, can all create lasting emotional distress. But new research suggests that nursing a grudge could put strain on our heart. Releasing that anger by forgiving the person who hurt us could help ease the burden.

The latest evidence comes from a study by researchers at Hope College in Michigan who asked volunteers to think about someone who had caused them pain. When the volunteers replayed in their minds the reasons they were angry and hurt, tests showed a spike in their blood pressure, heart rate, and muscle tension—the same psychological stress reactions that can trigger angina in people who have coronary artery disease and may even lead to artery damage in people who don't. But when those volunteers imagined themselves forgiving the person, tests showed a much less dramatic rise in signs of cardiovascular arousal.

No one has yet proved that people who tend to be more forgiving are less likely to develop heart disease, however—or that the act of forgiving someone will protect you from having a

heart attack. But when researchers at the University of Michigan surveyed more than 1,400 people in 2001, they did find that people who said they'd forgiven someone who'd hurt them also reported being in better overall health than those who had never forgiven anyone.

"To err is human, to forgive divine," as the eighteenth-century poet Alexander Pope wrote. That's still true today. In the University of Michigan study, only 52 percent of respondents said they had forgiven someone who had trespassed against them. But 75 percent believed that God had forgiven them for past wrongs.

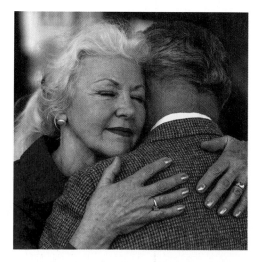

ire rising, count backward from 10, then take a few deep breaths, concentrating on letting your anger out each time you exhale.

4. Distract yourself. One of the simplest ways to banish nagging thoughts or sidestep anger is to put something positive in their place. Call a friend, put on a piece of music you love, take a hot bath, or lose yourself in a good book. Engaging in a hobby that absorbs your full concentration is a perfect antidote to stress. For many people, gardening can be particularly therapeutic.

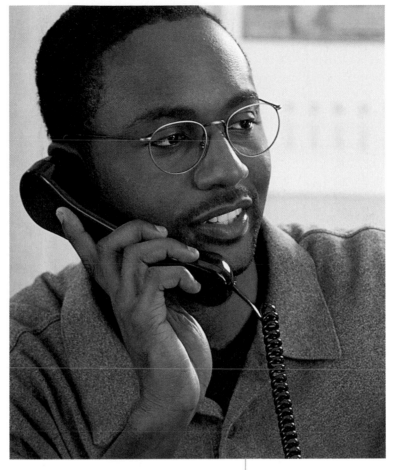

5. Get moving. Several studies have found that physical activity helps reduce stress and anxiety and may even be an effective remedy for mild to moderate depression. In a 1998 study in which 38 men and 35 women kept diaries of activity, mood, and stress, volunteers felt less stressed out on days when they were physically active than on those when they didn't exercise. Even when stressful events occurred, the participants felt less anxious on days when they were physically active. Exercise can also help ensure that you get a good night's sleep.

6. Call on a friend. Spending time with someone you like does more than take your mind off your troubles—it could save your life. Swedish researchers recently reported that people with a strong sense of social connection to other people were almost one-third less likely to die in the aftermath of having a heart attack than those who were socially isolated. If you don't have a circle of friends to turn to, try building one by, say, volunteering for a local charity or becoming involved with a local church.

Worth a Laugh

Looking for comic relief? Try one of these movies:

1. *A Fish Called Wanda* (1988)
2. *Annie Hall* (1977)
3. *Bringing Up Baby* (1938)
4. *Chicken Run* (2000)
5. *Dr. Strangelove* (1964)
6. *Duck Soup* (1933)
7. *Monty Python and the Holy Grail* (1975)
8. *Mrs. Doubtfire* (1993)
9. *Shrek* (2001)
10. *Some Like it Hot* (1959)
11. *The Apartment* (1960)
12. *The Princess Bride* (1987)
13. *The Sting* (1973)
14. *Tootsie* (1982)
15. *Toy Story* (1995)

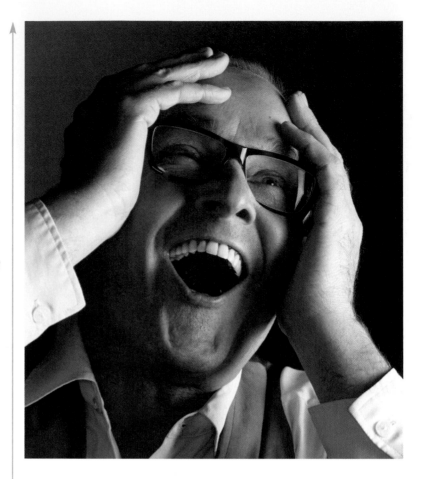

7. Have a good laugh. Laughter, it's said, is the best medicine. In fact, being able to laugh at life's stresses could be an antidote to heart disease. In a study published in 2001, researchers tested 300 volunteers' propensity to laugh at everyday situations, surprise events, or during encounters with friends. Those with a ready laugh were less likely to have coronary artery disease than those less apt to chuckle, the scientists found. Even among people with elevated blood pressure or cholesterol, the ability to laugh protected their hearts. If you can't seem to make light of the things going on in your own life, try renting a comedic movie or reading a comic novel.

The art of relaxation

You'd think relaxing would be easy. In fact, most of us have a hard time really emptying our minds and letting our bodies go limp. A little bit of practice can help.

There are all kinds of ways to quell worrisome thoughts and soothe the spirit. Some people are drawn to meditation. Others turn to prayer. The best method is simply one that allows you to find some quiet time away from the stresses of everyday life.

Relaxation is important not just to your emotional well-being but also to your health. Harvard University psychiatrist Herbert Benson was the first to study the physical effects of relaxation techniques such as meditation. His discoveries surprised much of the medical community. By meditating, he found, people could actually lower their blood pressure, slow their breathing, and reduce their body's oxygen consumption—controlling body functions previously thought to be entirely involuntary. In other words, while the body turns on the fight-or-flight response automatically, we can learn to turn it off, using what Benson calls the relaxation response. Eliciting the relaxation response is relatively simple. Just follow these steps.

1. Find a quiet place where you won't be disturbed. Sit in a comfortable position, one that will allow you to relax your body.

2. Close your eyes.

3. Breathe through your nose, concentrating on each breath. As you exhale, silently repeat a single word or short phrase, such as "peace" or "easy does it." Choose something soothing.

4. Continue repeating your word or phrase and concentrating on your breathing for 15 to 20 minutes. (Don't set an alarm, or you'll constantly be thinking about when it will go off. Have a watch or clock handy and open your eyes now and then to check the time.)

5. Sit quietly for a few minutes, first with your eyes closed and then with them open. Savor the way your body and mind feel.

Whatever method you choose to activate the relaxation response, don't defeat the purpose by worrying whether you're doing it correctly. The only measure of success is whether it helps you relax. And don't give up if you find bothersome thoughts intruding. Just put them gently aside and refocus your attention on your word or phrase. The more you practice your relaxation technique, the more effective it will be.

FAST FACT

In a 2000 study, men between ages 35 and 57 who took regular vacations were 30 percent less likely to die from heart disease during the nine-year study period than people who skipped their vacations.

163

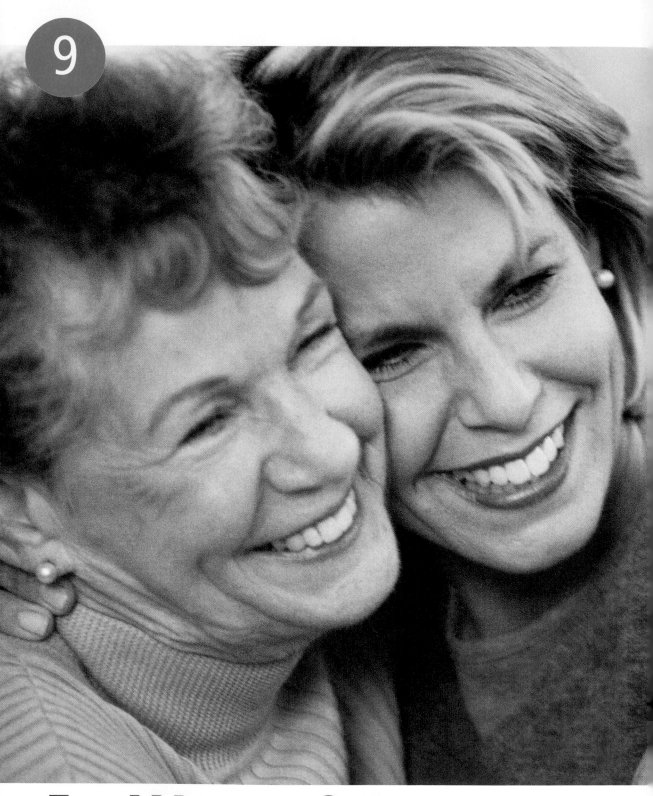

9

For Women Only

If you're like a lot of women, the most serious risk factor for heart disease you face is a false sense of security. Despite plenty of warnings to the contrary, many people still think of heart attacks primarily as a man's worry. That means they (and their physicians) are often slow to recognize the symptoms of trouble. The result: Women are dying of heart attacks that could have been prevented.

Heart disease is the leading cause of death for both sexes in the United States. Period. True, men begin having heart attacks earlier in life than women do, and until the age of 65 they suffer more of them. But once women have gone through menopause, their risk of coronary artery disease begins to climb rapidly, catching up with that of men by age 65.

Crossing the Gender Gap

When researchers first began to look closely at the risk of heart disease in women, they turned up some surprising—and deeply troubling—facts. Among them:

- Women with symptoms of coronary artery disease typically wait longer than men do before they see a doctor.
- They tend to be sicker when they are finally diagnosed.
- They are treated less aggressively than men when they complain of heart disease symptoms. They are less likely than men to be given angiograms, for instance, tests that use injected dye to create an image of coronary arteries.
- Women under age 50 are more likely than men to die of a first heart attack.

The biggest discrepancy between the sexes is the age when heart disease first shows up. Most women are protected until they go through menopause. The reasons aren't entirely clear, although many experts believe that high levels of the female hormone estrogen play a protective role. Estrogen decreases LDL ("bad" cholesterol) and boosts HDL ("good" cholesterol). It also raises levels of a chemical called tissue plasminogen activator, or TPA, which dissolves clots. Moreover, prior to menopause a woman's uterus

Once women have gone through menopause, their risk of coronary artery disease begins to climb rapidly.

165

churns out hormonelike chemicals called prostaglandins, which widen blood vessels and also help prevent clots from forming. All these effects are likely to ward off heart disease and heart attacks.

As estrogen levels dip after menopause, however, women's protection begins to vanish. By age 65 women have the same risk of coronary artery disease as men.

The fact that women develop heart disease later in life probably accounts for some of the differences in how the genders fare. Because women are an average 10 years older than men when they are diagnosed, they tend to have more complicating conditions, such as diabetes, high cholesterol, or elevated blood pressure—conditions that make heart disease more dangerous. In 1999 Yale University researchers analyzed data from 384,878 men and women who had suffered heart attacks. Almost 17 percent of the

WOMEN AND HEART DISEASE: TEST YOUR KNOWLEDGE

What you don't know about heart disease can hurt you. That's especially true for women, who may delay seeing a doctor because they think they aren't at serious risk. Test your knowledge by checking True or False. Correct answers follow.

❧ 1. The symptoms of a heart attack are always the same for women and men.
True ■ False ■

❧ 2. A heart attack is two times more likely to prove fatal for a woman under 50 than for a man of the same age.
True ■ False ■

❧ 3. Women are more likely to die of breast cancer than heart disease.
True ■ False ■

❧ 4. Among women, smoking causes just about as many deaths from heart disease as from lung cancer.
True ■ False ■

❧ 5. Estrogen replacement therapy has been proven to lower women's risk of dying from a heart attack.
True ■ False ■

❧ 6. Estrogen replacement therapy has been linked to increased risk of breast cancer.
True ■ False ■

❧ 7. Diabetes poses a more serious risk to a woman's heart than to a man's.
True ■ False ■

❧ 8. Low levels of "good" cholesterol pose a more serious risk to women than to men.
True ■ False ■

❧ 9. After age 65 a woman's blood pressure is typically higher than a man's.
True ■ False ■

Answers:

1. False	4. True	7. True
2. True	5. False	8. True
3. False	6. True	9. True

166

women died while hospitalized compared with only 11.5 percent of the men. But when the researchers accounted for the effects of age, the difference in death rates all but disappeared.

There was one exception, however. And it's a worrisome one. Women under 50 who suffered a heart attack were twice as likely to die from it as were men of the same age. The younger that women were at the time of their first heart attack, the more likely it was to be fatal.

Why remains a mystery. The hazards of heart disease may be more serious in females than males simply because women's bodies—including their hearts and blood vessels—are smaller. Cholesterol buildup may be more dangerous in smaller arteries than in larger ones. Similarly, coronary artery disease may be harder on a small heart than on a larger one.

Key Finding

Many women still don't take the threat of heart disease seriously, according to results from a telephone survey of 1,000 people conducted by New York-Presbyterian Hospital. Although half of American women die of heart disease or stroke, only 8 percent of those polled identified either of these problems as their greatest health worry. Only one in three realized that heart disease is the leading cause of death among women. Those under age 44 were more likely to put breast cancer in the top spot. Perhaps most worrisome of all, 70 percent of the women polled said they had never talked to their doctors about heart disease or how to prevent it.

But these differences don't explain all the seeming inequities between the sexes. The fact is, some doctors may be less likely to suspect heart disease in a female patient—especially those under 60. As a result, they may be less likely to order diagnostic tests such as stress tests or angiograms. One recent study found that angiograms were performed on 59 percent of men with symptoms of coronary artery disease compared with only 53 percent of women. (Some critics argue that angiograms are actually performed too often on men—not less often than necessary on women. But since these tests are used to screen people who may need bypasses or other surgery, the difference in rates does suggest that some women aren't getting the care they need.) And the sad fact is that many younger women don't give their risk of heart disease a thought. At almost any age, women tend to be more preoccupied with breast cancer risk, even though the danger to their hearts is far more significant.

The bottom line: Take the risk of heart disease seriously, and learn to recognize the symptoms of heart attack. If you've already been diagnosed with coronary artery disease, take charge of your medical care by asking your doctor to discuss all the treatment options. If you're not comfortable with the advice and information you're given, get a second opinion.

Understanding a Woman's Risks

Although age difference is the most important distinction between the genders when it comes to heart disease, there are others. For instance, some risk factors, like diabetes, pose a more serious danger to women than to men. Also, when men first develop symptoms of heart disease, they typically have one or two risk factors. Women are more likely to have multiple risk factors that, together, compound the danger. More women than men tend to be obese and have both high blood pressure and elevated cholesterol, for example. Being overweight and having diabetes also seem to go hand in hand for many women.

Understanding the special concerns women face can help you fine-tune your strategy for staying healthy. Here's what you need to know.

Diabetes. Diabetes may be more dangerous to a woman's heart than a man's, research suggests. Three out of four people with diabetes will end up dying of some form of cardiovascular disease. But while having diabetes increases a man's risk of heart disease by two- to threefold, a woman's jumps by as much as sevenfold. This may be because in women diabetes often occurs in the presence of other cardiovascular risk factors, such as obesity, physical inactivity, high blood pressure, and elevated cholesterol. Still, many researchers are now convinced that diabetes, especially for women, is one of the most serious risk factors for heart disease.

Blood pressure. High blood pressure increases heart disease risk in both men and women, but the problem may be more serious in women. By the time women reach age 55, more than half have blood pressure high enough to put

FAST FACT

Contrary to the myth that it's a man's problem, cardiovascular disease (including heart attack and stroke) actually kills 43,000 more women than men in the United States each year.

Symptoms of Their Own?

Are the symptoms of heart attack different in men than women? You would think so, reading some popular books and websites devoted to women's health. But focusing on differences, some experts say, could be doing women more harm than good.

Here's why. While it's true that a percentage of women, particularly those on the young side, experience atypical symptoms (instead of pain or pressure in their chests, they may feel only nausea or severe indigestion, along with shortness of breath, for instance), the number is quite small. In the overwhelming majority, the same alarm sounds: pain or pressure in the middle of the chest, often radiating out down the left arm, accompanied by sweating, nausea, or shortness of breath.

By emphasizing gender differences in heart attack symptoms, critics say, some information resources may actually make women less alert to the most common indications of trouble.

For middle-age and older women, the advice is simple: If you experience chest pain or pressure and/or shortness of breath especially during physical activity or emotional stress, call your doctor or dial 911 and chew an aspirin. Don't wait. Studies show that women tend to put off seeing a doctor longer than men when the symptoms of coronary artery disease appear. That delay, for some, can prove fatal.

---

them in the cross hairs of danger. After age 65, women typically have higher blood pressure than men. The problem is more severe among African-American women.

Cholesterol. Elevated LDL is dangerous for both sexes. But from age 55 on, women's LDL levels tend to be higher than men's. Women may also be at greater risk when their levels of good cholesterol, or HDL, dip low. In one recent study, low HDL was one of the most significant signals of increased heart disease risk in women, though not in men. (Elevated LDL appears to pose more danger in men.) What's more, women seem to need slightly more HDL to ward off heart disease. The official guidelines for both sexes advise maintaining an HDL level of 40 mg/dL, but some studies show that women require at least 45 mg/dL for protection.

Smoking. Although smoking rates are declining among both sexes, the rate of decline is lower in women. Why? One reason may be that women have a harder time kicking the habit. Yet they may be at greater risk from smoking. In a 1999 study by Italian scientists, women who smoked were more than four times more likely to suffer a heart attack; men's risk was just over threefold higher.

Using the Pill. Alarms sounded a few years ago when researchers linked oral contraceptives with a greatly increased risk

LIFESAVING INSIGHTS FROM AMERICA'S NURSES

In 1976 millions of women around the country were using oral contraceptives—potent drugs whose long-term effects had never been studied. To uncover any hidden health dangers, researchers at Harvard University contacted 170,000 nurses, asking them to fill out a questionnaire. Nurses were chosen in part because their medical expertise would make it easy for them to answer the brief but technical questions accurately. Some 122,000 people responded. And the Nurses' Health Study was born.

Recognizing that the nurses offered an unprecedented opportunity to study many aspects of women's health, the Harvard team began collecting more and more detailed information—about everything from smoking and hormone use to diet and exercise. Between 1982 and 1984 the study subjects even submitted 68,000 sets of toenail samples, which were used to analyze nutrient content in the diet. Even today, more than 25 years after the study started, 90 percent of the questionnaires sent out every two years are filled in and returned.

Over that time, scientists have gained lifesaving insights into heart disease among women. Highlights include:

■ **The risks of being overweight.** Nurses who gained 55 pounds over the course of the study period had more than a fivefold risk of developing high blood pressure. Overweight nurses who lost weight lowered their risk by 25 percent.

■ **The benefits of physical activity.** Walking at a pace of more than three miles an hour for at least one hour a week lowered the risk of stroke by about 30 percent. Walking three or more hours a week at a brisk pace slashed heart disease risk by 35 percent.

■ **The importance of whole grains.** Women who ate at least one serving of whole grains a day cut their risk of ischemic stroke by 30 to 40 percent and their risk of diabetes by 25 percent.

■ **The dangers of smoking.** Heart disease is three times more prevalent among women who smoke than nonsmokers.

■ **The risks of refined carbohydrates.** Women whose diets were top-heavy with sugars and other highly refined carbohydrates had a two and a half times higher risk of heart disease than women who ate the lowest amounts of such foods.

■ **A warning for snorers.** Women who reported snoring were more than twice as likely as those who didn't snore to develop cardiovascular disease.

■ **The protective effects of fiber.** Findings showed that eating one serving of a high-fiber breakfast cereal each day can cut heart disease risk by as much as 35 percent.

of heart attack. According to several studies, women on the pill were three to four times more likely to have a heart attack. But these numbers may not be as scary as they seem. For starters, during childbearing years the overall risk of heart attack is very low, so the actual number of attacks linked to birth control pills is quite small. And newer oral contraceptives, which contain far less estrogen than earlier versions, have been shown to pose virtually no

Key Finding

Women are at greater risk of sudden and serious heart attacks during certain times of the month according to a small study of premenopausal women with heart disease symptoms. Among the 28 women studied, 20 reported developing heart-related problems within five days of beginning their periods, when estrogen is at its lowest ebb.

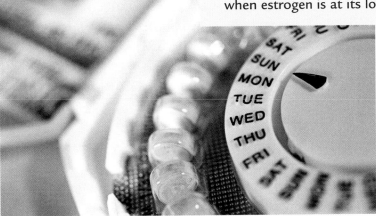

risk. There is one exception. A 2001 study by researchers from Boston University School of Medicine found that the incidence of heart attacks was as much as 39 times higher than normal among heavy smokers on the pill than among nonsmokers on the pill.

Being inactive and overweight. More than 6 out of 10 American women barely get any exercise at all. And that number is rising, researchers say. What a pity, since studies show that being sedentary more than doubles a woman's risk of dying from a heart attack. Lack of exercise is also a factor in the growing number of people who are overweight. Carrying excess pounds raises heart disease risk for both men and women, but research suggests it increases it more for women. One long-term study of 116,000 women found that almost 40 percent of coronary heart disease was attributable to being overweight.

The bottom line: Making heart healthy lifestyle changes may be even more important for women than it is for men, since

4

Things to Know About ERT

1

ERT comes in many different forms.
Replacement estrogen can be delivered via pills, patches, creams, and other methods. If you're considering ERT, talk to your doctor about the best choice for you.

2

Many women experience side effects.
Although ERT eases some symptoms associated with menopause, it can also cause bloating, breast tenderness, cramping, spotting, or a return to monthly periods.

3

Dietary estrogens may offer protection.
Some studies have shown that estrogen-like substances, called phytoestrogens, found in soy and other plant foods may lower heart disease risk, although the evidence is controversial.

4

New dangers may lurk.
In a study published in 2001, researchers at the American Cancer Society found an increased risk of ovarian cancer in women who had taken ERT.

eating a nutritious diet and getting a moderate dose of exercise on most days of the week are the most effective ways to keep many of these threats under control.

The Estrogen Question

To take estrogen or not to take estrogen. For millions of post-menopausal women, the issue of heart disease has come down to this one troubling question. At first, estrogen promised to be a virtual fountain of youth, heading off not only heart disease but also many other age-related conditions. Then came word that estrogen replacement therapy (ERT) can raise a woman's risk of breast cancer—and suddenly the potential benefits had to be weighed against a scary risk. Now, new findings further complicate the issue. While recent studies have shown that ERT protects older women from age-related memory loss and also helps ward off bone loss, it seems the heart disease prevention power of ERT may not be nearly as certain as researchers once hoped.

From high hopes to nagging worries

It's easy to understand why cardiologists thought that taking estrogen might protect women's hearts. After all, as levels of the hormone fall in menopause, heart disease risk climbs in lockstep. Taking synthetic estrogen should, by all rights, extend the protection afforded by the natural hormone.

And indeed, early research findings augured well. Between 1987 and 1998 dozens of studies showed that women who took estrogen after menopause had lower rates of coronary artery disease than those who didn't. In 1996, for instance, results from the Nurses' Health Study found that women receiving estrogen were about half as likely as those not taking the hormone to develop the disease. Another study found that angina and heart attacks occurred 80 percent less often in postmenopausal women on ERT.

Most of these studies were what researchers call observational studies. In other words, scientists simply observed large groups of women, including some who'd decided to take ERT. The trouble with such studies is that women who decide to take ERT may differ in other ways from those who don't. They may eat healthier diets, for instance, or get more exercise. The way around this problem is to do randomized studies, in which women are randomly assigned to receive estrogen or a dummy pill and then followed to see how they fare. Randomized trials are considered the gold standard of medical research.

To almost everyone's surprise, the results of such studies for ERT have been disappointing. The first such study was the Heart and Estrogen/Progestin Replacement Study, or HERS, which involved 2,763 women with coronary artery disease. Some volunteers were put on a combination of estrogen and progestin; others were given a placebo. Four years later, tests showed that women on ERT had LDL ("bad" cholesterol) levels 11 percent lower and HDL ("good" cholesterol) levels 10 percent higher than women on the dummy pills—strong evidence that estrogen should be lowering their risk. Yet the women on ERT were just as likely to have a heart attack during the four years of the study. In fact, during the first year of the study, women in the ERT group were actually more likely to suffer angina or a heart attack. After the first year, however, that added risk disappeared; by the end of the study, researchers began to see evidence of a small benefit to women on ERT.

LOOKING AHEAD
Safer estrogen on the horizon

New forms of estrogen replacement therapy could help doctors eliminate the drawbacks of estrogen and zero in on certain benefits. The new forms are called selective estrogen receptor modulators, or SERMS. They are designed to stimulate only certain tissues, leaving others undisturbed. One SERM under investigation, called raloxifene (brand name Evista), stimulates bone growth but leaves breast cells alone. Researchers hope to find SERMs that will offer the cardiovascular and bone protection of natural estrogen while blocking its cancer-stimulating effects.

Results from another major study, called Estrogen Replacement and Atherosclerosis, further undermined hopes for ERT. Scientists randomly divided women into three groups. Those in the first received estrogen alone. Those in the second received estrogen and progestin. Women in the third were given placebos. In all three groups, the progress of coronary artery disease, evidenced by angiograms, was the same.

Meanwhile, estrogen's effect on breast cancer risk wasn't going away. In a report from the Nurses' Health Study published in 2000, for example, scientists compared breast cancer risk in more than 46,000 women interviewed between 1973 and 1995. Women who were currently using ERT—or had used it sometime during the previous four years—were 20 to 40 percent more likely to develop breast cancer than those not on therapy.

> "There are plenty of ways to prevent heart disease that are safer and more certain than estrogen replacement therapy."

What's a woman to do?

In the wake of the new data, many cardiologists have altered their advice to women. Even the American Heart Association has withdrawn its recommendation that women with heart disease consider ERT. The results of ongoing studies may shed more light on the picture. But for now, here's what most experts say.

If you've been diagnosed with coronary artery disease, there's little evidence that starting ERT will help you ward off a heart attack or slow the progress of the disease. And because studies show an increased risk of heart attacks during the first year on ERT, most experts now think the risks outweigh the benefits.

If you're healthy but want to reduce your risk of heart disease, reliable advice is harder to come by. So far, all randomized studies have looked at women who already have heart disease. But some experts think ERT may prevent heart disease in healthy women. Several studies are under way to answer the question; results are several years away. Meanwhile, there are more reliable ways to protect yourself, including exercise and a healthier diet.

What if you're currently on ERT? Should you stop? Talk to your doctor. If you've been on ERT for more than a year without any problem, you're probably past the period of increased heart attack risk. There's preliminary evidence that ERT begins to offer some heart-disease protection after the first year. Of course, you still have to wrestle with the issue of breast cancer. If the disease runs in your family, ERT may not be worth the added risk.

In reality, most women start using ERT to ease the symptoms of menopause, such as hot flashes. And the majority stop taking it within the first year because they don't like the side effects.

Tried-and-true tactics

Luckily, there are plenty of ways to prevent heart disease that are safer and more certain than estrogen replacement therapy. Recent findings from the Nurses' Health Study show how powerful they can be. During a 15-year period, scientists counted 1,128 heart attacks in a group of more than 84,000 women. Of those heart attacks, 82 percent, the researchers concluded, could have been prevented if the women had followed basic heart disease prevention strategies. Those who most closely followed the familiar advice—to give up smoking, exercise at least 30 minutes per day, and eat a high-fiber diet low in saturated fats and trans fats—were 80 percent less likely than the others to develop heart disease.

REAL PEOPLE, REAL WISDOM

Warnings You Shouldn't Ignore

That's odd, Sheila Schrier remembers thinking. Starting her regular workout on the treadmill at the fitness club, she felt unusually tired for the first five minutes. The feeling passed, though, and she didn't give it a second thought. She certainly never worried about her heart.

"My husband had had bypass surgery a few years before, and he'd had such a hard time of it," says Schrier, 64. "I was so preoccupied with his health that I never stopped to worry about my own. I knew that women get heart disease, but somehow I never really thought that could mean me."

When she experienced the same tiredness the next time she used the treadmill, however, Schrier thought she'd better see her doctor. And it's a good thing she did. An angiogram showed that one of her coronary arteries was almost 90 percent blocked.

"If I had a dollar for every time someone said, 'How could this happen to you?' I'd be a millionaire," she says now with a laugh. Slender and in tip-top shape, Schrier is the director of a fitness center that specializes in cardiac rehabilitation programs. Before her diagnosis, she taught classes in water aerobics and worked out several times a week. She had always eaten a healthy diet. Her cholesterol levels were normal. And though she'd developed borderline high blood pressure after menopause, she was taking a drug that brought it under control.

Her only real risk factor was a family history of heart disease: Both her parents died of heart attacks. "But they both smoked. They ate terrible diets. I was sure that by living a healthy life I'd be able to avoid that," explains Schrier.

In fact, she did avoid a heart attack—by getting to the doctor in time, before the blockage cut off blood flow entirely. When an attempt to open up the blocked artery through angioplasty failed, Schrier underwent a coronary bypass, in which a new blood vessel, transplanted from another part of the body, is connected to supply the heart. Two months after the operation, she started a rehabilitation program—as a patient this time. "It wasn't easy," she remembers. "After the surgery, I was completely incapacitated. There were moments when I would suddenly feel panicky. It takes a while to get your energy back, and your confidence."

A year later, she's back to work and even back to doing her own workouts, although not quite as strenuously as before. "One thing I've come away from the experience realizing is how important it is to listen to your body," she says. "I think a lot of times when a woman complains about how she's feeling, there's a tendency for doctors to say, 'Oh, it's all in her head.' Fortunately, when something didn't feel quite right to me, I went to the doctor. I insisted that the tests be done. That may very well have saved my life."

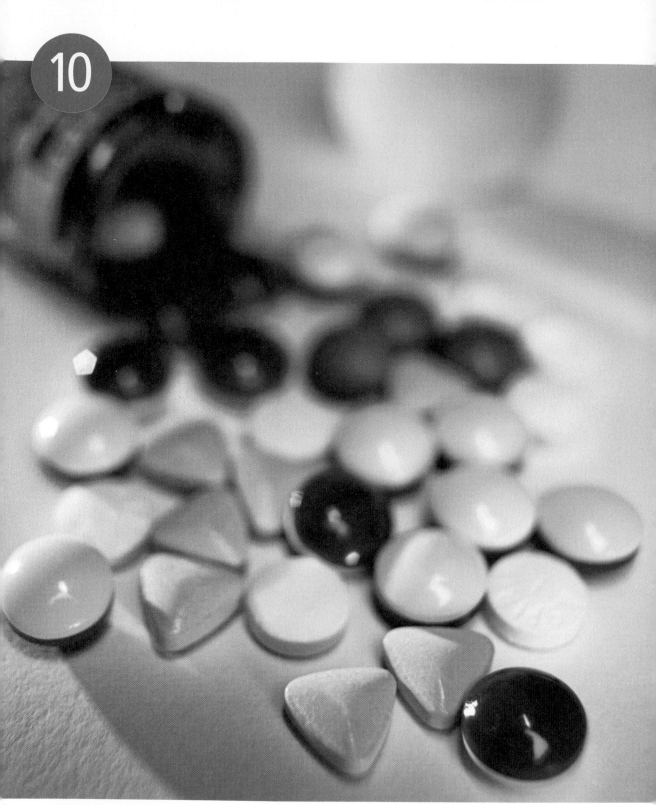

10

Taking Your Medicine

Researchers haven't yet devised a pill to cure heart disease, but they've scored some very important victories. If you're at risk for heart disease but are still healthy, the latest medicines can help you stay that way. If you've been diagnosed with coronary artery disease, new drugs can increase blood flow and ease the burden on your heart. Even during a heart attack, that old medicine-cabinet standby, aspirin, has been proven to help limit the damage to the heart. Meanwhile, sophisticated "super aspirins" have come along that offer even more powerful heart protection.

Surprisingly, one of the biggest challenges cardiologists now face is getting people to take their medicines. Failure to use drugs as directed is a big and growing problem. The more effective a heart disease medication is, the more important it is to take it as prescribed. Fall short, and you could be shortchanging yourself on lifesaving benefits.

Taking the Risk Out of Risk Factors

One of the biggest advances in recent years has been the development of new drugs for conditions that increase heart disease risk, such as elevated cholesterol and high blood pressure. In people with elevated cholesterol, for instance, the latest generation of cholesterol-lowering drugs was recently shown to slash the risk of heart attacks by 30 percent. An estimated 50,000 heart disease deaths could be prevented each year in the United States alone, experts say, if everyone with cholesterol levels in the danger zone were taking them. Even people with only moderately elevated cholesterol levels could benefit from these medications, recent evidence suggests. If that's true, half of all Americans might do well to begin drug therapy. Yet barely 35 percent of those who could most benefit from these medications are taking them.

Why? Cost is certainly one reason. Another is lack of knowledge. There are still plenty of people out there who don't know

In people with elevated cholesterol, the latest generation of cholesterol-lowering drugs was recently shown to slash the risk of heart attacks by 30 percent.

that their cholesterol levels are too high. Critics fault doctors for not being aggressive enough in testing their patients or prescribing the medications. Even when physicians prescribe the drugs, though, many people don't follow doctors' orders. Studies show that as many as half of patients prescribed statin drugs like Lipitor (atorvastatin) stop taking them within the first year. The same problems limit the effectiveness of other potentially lifesaving drugs, including those that control blood pressure and diabetes.

The cholesterol tamers

Moderately elevated cholesterol can often be brought under control with a healthier diet that's low in saturated fat and abundant in high-fiber foods. But not everyone's cholesterol responds to dietary changes. Some people have cholesterol so high that even the best diet can't bring it back down to earth. Fortunately, a variety of medications can do the trick safely and effectively. Here's how the leading drugs stack up.

Statins (HMG-CoA reductase inhibitors). The newest cholesterol-fighting medications, statins lower cholesterol levels by blocking an enzyme in the body that is needed to make cholesterol. Statins reduce both LDL cholesterol and triglyceride levels and raise HDL levels slightly.

When scientists analyzed data from five large trials involving more than 30,000 patients, statins were found to reduce total cholesterol by an average of 20 percent and LDL cholesterol by 28 percent. Triglycerides fell by 13 percent. HDL cholesterol rose by

ARE STATINS SAFE?

If you're taking a cholesterol-lowering statin, chances are you've heard the news that one such drug, sold under the name Baycol (cerivastatin), was yanked from the market. In August 2001 the FDA announced that the drug's manufacturer was voluntarily withdrawing the medication after 31 Americans taking it died due to rhabdomyolysis, a severe problem that results in the breakdown of muscle cells. Other statins have also been associated with rhabdomyolysis, but the problem is exceedingly rare among users of these forms of the drug. Baycol was withdrawn only when reports suggested a higher risk to users. Experts say the very real benefits of cholesterol-lowering statins—including a dramatically reduced threat of heart attacks—far outweigh the very small dangers.

about 5 percent. All four changes help lower the risk of heart disease and heart attacks.

Now that experts have revised the recommended levels of LDL and HDL cholesterol, you may be a candidate for statin drugs even if you weren't before. According to the American Heart Association, you're a candidate for drug therapy if:

- You're at very low risk of coronary artery disease, but your LDL cholesterol is 190 mg/dL or higher
- You have two or more risk factors for coronary artery disease, and your LDL cholesterol is 160 mg/dL or higher
- You have coronary artery disease, and your LDL cholesterol is 130 mg/dL or higher

Key Finding

Taking a statin drug? You may want to think twice before scooping up antioxidant supplements like vitamins C and E. In a study published in November 2001 in *The New England Journal of Medicine*, researchers found that antioxidants blunted the effectiveness of the statin drug Zocor (simvastatin) in people who were also taking niacin. The scientists measured the rate of atherosclerosis in 160 patients. Those taking the two drugs saw their blockages decrease slightly. Patients who added antioxidants saw theirs increase by .7 percent.

Because statins are processed in the liver, doctors recommend periodic blood tests to check how your liver is functioning. Examples of statin drugs include Lipitor (atorvastatin), Mevacor (lovastatin), Zocor (simvastatin), and Pravachol (pravastatin). Not all insurance plans cover all these drugs. And prices vary widely. If money is an issue, ask your doctor whether you can switch to a cheaper version.

Bile acid sequestrants. Like statin drugs, bile acid sequestrants help the body get rid of LDL cholesterol. Studies show that these drugs lower LDL levels by about 10 to 20 percent. Bile acid sequestrants usually come in a powder that has to be mixed with water or juice. Examples include Questran (cholestyramine) and Colestid (colestipol hydrochloride).

Niacin (nicotinic acid). Niacin, a form of B vitamin, was one of the first cholesterol drugs, and doctors still prescribe it, especially for patients with low levels of "good" cholesterol. The reason: It's one of the only drugs that significantly boosts HDL. On average, niacin reduces LDL cholesterol by 10 to 20 percent, decreases triglycerides by 20 to 50 percent, and boosts HDL by 15 to 35 percent. The only reason doctors don't prescribe niacin more often is that it can cause uncomfortable side effects, including nausea, indigestion, gas, vomiting, and diarrhea, as well as liver problems, when people take too much too quickly. Doctors usually start with a low dose and gradually increase it to effective levels to give the body time to get used to it. Brand names for niacin include Niacor and Nicolar.

The blood pressure brigade

Lowering your blood pressure by even a few points can make a big difference to your health. One recent study showed that bringing diastolic blood pressure (the bottom number) down just 6 mm/Hg reduced death from heart attacks by 14 percent and strokes by 42 percent. For some people, exercise and a low-salt, high-fiber diet does the trick. If not, there are drugs that can safely rein in elevated blood pressure. The most common categories include:

Diuretics. Sometimes called water pills, diuretics work in the kidney, flushing extra water and sodium out of the body and, thus, reducing the amount of fluid in the blood. One of the most commonly prescribed is a one-a-day pill that contains hydrochlorothiazide, marketed under a variety of brand names, including Oretic, Esidrix, and HydroDIURIL.

Beta-blockers. Beta-blockers reduce blood pressure by blocking nerve impulses to the heart and blood vessels, making the heart beat more slowly and with less force. Beta-blockers are sometimes used to restore normal heartbeat rhythm to people with some types of arrhythmias. Examples include Inderal (propranolol), Lopressor (metoprolol), and Levatol (penbutolol).

Alpha-blockers. Alpha-blockers reduce another form of nerve impulse to blood vessels, allowing blood to flow through more easily and, thus, reducing blood pressure. Examples include Cardura (doxazosin) and Hytrin (terazosin).

Alpha-beta-blockers. This combined drug relaxes blood vessels and slows heartbeat. The result: Less blood is pumped through vessels, and blood pressure falls. One commonly prescribed alpha-beta-blocker is Normodyne (labetalol).

ACE inhibitors. ACE (angiotensin-converting enzyme) inhibitors block the production of a hormone called angiotensin II that causes blood vessels to narrow. With less of the hormone in the body, blood vessels remain open, and blood pressure falls. Examples include Capoten (captopril) and Vasotec (enalapril).

FAST FACT

Grapefruit and grapefruit juice can interact with certain heart medications. If you're a grapefruit fan, tell your doctor.

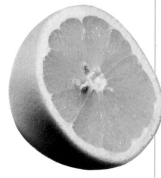

Angiotensin receptor blockers. A new alternative to ACE inhibitors, ARBs directly block the hormone angiotensin II from binding to blood vessels and, thus, constricting them. Some patients experience fewer side effects with angiotensin receptor blockers than with ACE inhibitors. Examples include Avapro (irbesartan) and Diovan (valsartan).

Vasodilators. These drugs work directly on the muscles in blood vessel walls, relaxing them. As blood flows more easily, pressure drops. Examples of vasodilators are Apresoline (hydralazine) and Loniten (minoxidil).

Don't be surprised if your doctor prescribes two or more blood pressure medications. Many of these drugs work best in combination. And you may find that your physician has to tinker with the combination to get it just right—or change it over time as your blood pressure changes. It sometimes takes a little while for doctors to hit on just the right prescription. If you experience symptoms like dizziness or coughing (a potential side effect of ACE inhibitors), be sure to mention them to your doctor.

Easing the Burden on Ailing Hearts

If you've already been diagnosed with coronary artery disease, several drugs can help ease the strain on your heart and relieve angina, the chest pain or pressure that occurs when blocked coronary arteries make it hard for the heart to get the oxygenated blood it needs.

Angina medications work by increasing blood flow through obstructed arteries or by reducing the heart muscle's need for oxygen, or both. If you have only mild angina or experience the symptoms only now and then, your doctor may recommend a drug to take when you feel the problem coming on. If you experience angina regularly, your doctor may recommend a drug that you take every day. Medications to treat angina include:

Nitrates (nitroglycerin). Nitrates have been used for more than a century to relieve angina, and they are still among the most common drugs prescribed. They work by widening blood vessels, making it easier for oxygenated blood to reach the heart. Nitrates come in tablet, ointment, spray, or patch

TROUBLESHOOTING TIP

If you have angina, keep a bottle of nitroglycerin pills or spray on hand in case you experience chest pain. But pay attention to the expiration date. Nitroglycerin loses its effectiveness six weeks after the bottle has been opened. The drug is sensitive to light and moisture, so don't leave the container in a sunny place and don't store it in the bathroom or refrigerator.

form. Usually the tablets are dissolved under your tongue or between lip and gum so the active ingredients reach the bloodstream rapidly. The spray is also administered under the tongue.

Nitrates can be used when you are having an angina episode or if you are about to encounter a situation that typically triggers one, such as physical activity or a stressful event. The drugs work very quickly, usually within three to five minutes. In some cases you may need to take more than one pill. If the pain hasn't gone away after 15 minutes, call an ambulance to drive you to the nearest emergency room.

Calcium channel blockers. Calcium channel blockers interrupt the ability of calcium molecules to enter muscle cells in the heart and blood vessels. The result: Heart rate slows, and the strength of the contractions diminishes, reducing the heart's oxy-

HOT TOPIC

Taking a Pill vs. Making a Change

With all the hoopla over the latest cholesterol-lowering drugs, it's easy to wonder what ever happened to making lifestyle changes like getting more exercise and eating a healthier diet. Weren't they supposed to rein in runaway cholesterol and keep blood pressure from going through the roof?

Indeed, many experts worry that Americans may rely too much on pharmaceuticals and not enough on leading healthier lives. Reports suggest that some people taking medications like statins actually begin to ignore advice about healthy eating, convinced that the drugs will make up for the shortcomings of their diets.

The truth is, keeping to a healthy diet and getting plenty of exercise are still the best proven ways to reduce your chances of having a heart attack. Drugs that improve cholesterol levels or tame high blood pressure are only a second line of defense, when lifestyle changes don't work. But there's plenty of evidence that they usually do. One study found that volunteers dropped their LDL levels by a whopping 33 percent by following a diet low in saturated fat and loaded with fruit and vegetables. A combination of exercise and a high-fiber, low-fat diet has been shown to bring moderately elevated blood pressure back down into the safe zone—without the help of any drugs.

Not surprisingly, however, people in the real world don't usually do as well making lifestyle changes as do volunteers in tightly controlled studies. As much as no one likes to admit it, it's easier for some people to pop a pill than to turn their eating and exercise habits around.

Remember: Pills never replace the need to make lifestyle changes. Even if you do end up having to take drugs for cholesterol or blood pressure, it's still important to help your medicine along. The more you improve your numbers through diet and exercise, the less medication you'll need. And the healthier your heart will be, since diet and exercise provide a host of other benefits that no pill can offer.

gen needs. Calcium channel blockers also widen blood vessels and lower blood pressure, making it easier for the heart to pump blood through the body. Examples include Cardizem (diltiazem), DynaCirc (isradipine), and Procardia (nifedipine).

Beta-blockers. The same drugs that are used to lower blood pressure can also help treat angina. Beta-blockers slow the heartbeat and reduce blood pressure, particularly during physical activity, making it possible for people with angina to exert themselves more before developing chest pain. These drugs have been shown to cut the risk of having a second heart attack in half and to lower cardiac mortality rates by 20 percent.

TROUBLESHOOTING TIP

Bad cold? If you have hypertension or are taking a blood pressure medication, talk to your doctor before you take an over-the-counter decongestant. Recent studies show that decongestants can interfere with blood pressure drugs and raise your pressure. A new generation of decongestant-free medications are available over the counter to ease the symptoms of colds or allergies. Ask your pharmacist.

An Aspirin a Day?

Talk about a wonder drug! After years of being used to ease aches and pains, startling findings showed that aspirin offers powerful protection against heart attacks. Aspirin works by thinning the blood so that clots can't form as easily.

The best evidence for aspirin's heart benefits is in people already diagnosed with coronary artery disease. If you've had a heart attack, taking aspirin will help prevent the formation of new blood clots that might lead to a second attack. If you've had coronary bypass surgery, taking aspirin will lower the chances that your new arteries will become blocked with clots. If you're having a heart attack, putting an aspirin under your tongue rushes anticlotting substances into the bloodstream that could dissolve the clot and dramatically reduce the risk of heart muscle damage.

But what if you don't have heart problems? Can aspirin lower your risk of developing coronary artery disease? The evidence isn't clear. When Harvard University researchers looked at 22,000 male physicians, they found that men who took one aspirin every other day had 44 percent fewer heart attacks. The benefits were so dramatic that the study was interrupted early so the results could be reported and all the volunteers in the study advised of aspirin's potential benefits.

But a similar study in Britain, which also followed physicians, found no such evidence that aspirin offered any protection.

For now, most experts do not recommend that people free of heart disease take aspirin to lower their risk—partly because the evidence of benefits is uncertain and partly because taking aspirin daily or even every other day can irritate the stomach lining and cause gastrointestinal bleeding.

If you have heart disease, ask your doctor about taking aspirin. The latest evidence suggests that a very small dose, just 81 milligrams—roughly one-quarter the amount in a standard adult tablet—is enough to protect your heart. So, most cardiologists recommend taking a baby aspirin, which contains about one-fourth the adult dose. Don't start popping pills on your own, however. Aspirin can cause problems if you're already taking a blood-thinning medication or if you have asthma.

TROUBLESHOOTING TIP

If you're taking aspirin to prevent a heart attack, what should you take for pain? Not ibuprofen (the pain reliever found in Advil and Motrin). In a 2001 study, University of Pennsylvania researchers found that aspirin loses 90 to 98 percent of its blood-thinning power when combined with ibuprofen. Scientists think that ibuprofen blocks up a channel in a clotting enzyme, preventing aspirin from reaching its target. Acetaminophen (such as Tylenol) is a better choice.

Beyond aspirin

New drugs even more powerful than aspirin have come along that can break up life-threatening blood clots and help prevent new ones from forming. Every year, thousands of people survive heart attacks that might have been fatal, thanks to such medications. The drugs are also prescribed after procedures such as angioplasty and bypass surgery to ward off new blockages. Here are the main types.

Thrombolytics. Usually administered intravenously during a heart attack, these drugs dissolve clots in arteries that supply both the lungs and the heart. In about 80 percent of heart attack patients who are given a thrombolytic drug within two hours after symptoms start, blood flow is restored. Examples include Kabikinase (streptokinase) and Eminase (anistreplase).

Anticoagulants. As the name suggests, anticoagulants help prevent blood from coagulating, or clotting. They work by reducing the amount of protein in the blood that is involved in clotting. Some anticoagulants are administered by injection, others in pill form. They are usually prescribed after a heart attack or an angioplasty to reduce the chances of new clots forming. They are sometimes also used to prevent clots in people with heart failure. (A weak pumping action means sluggish blood flow, which increases the likelihood of clots.) Examples include Coumadin (warfarin) and Calciparin (heparin). If you're taking a blood thinner, talk to your doctor before taking aspirin, vitamin E, or fish oil, all of which also thin the blood.

Super aspirins. These drugs work like aspirins do—by inhibiting the function of platelets, which are blood cells involved in clotting. One such drug, recently approved by the FDA, is Aggrastat (tirofiban hydrochloride). It's modeled on a venom used by the African saw-scaled viper. The venom contains a protein that prevents platelets in the blood from clumping together, causing the victim to bleed to death. Aggrastat is often prescribed for patients with unstable angina. Cardiologists at McMasters University in Canada recently tested another super aspirin, called Plavix (clopidogrel bisulfate). In patients with angina, the drug proved just as effective as angioplasty at reopening clogged arteries. Like anticoagulants, super aspirins are usually prescribed to patients who have had a heart attack or undergone an angioplasty or angiogram.

LOOKING AHEAD
Gene therapy for heart attack protection

Intensive research is under way to understand the genetic basis of heart disease—research that could yield new treatments in the form of gene therapy. In a preliminary study, scientists at the University of Arkansas recently tested a genetic approach to limiting heart muscle damage during heart attacks. When blood supply to the heart is cut off, blood levels of a protein called angiotensin-converting enzyme, or ACE, rise steeply. This worsens heart muscle damage. To counter the destructive effect, researchers designed a strand of DNA that attaches to the gene that controls the production of ACE protein, blocking it. In animal studies this approach was shown to protect the hearts of rats during heart attacks. Trials in humans are the next step.

Good Drugs, Bad Patients

While researchers have been able to create dozens of lifesaving heart medications, they haven't found a way to do something much more basic but equally important: get patients to take their medicine as directed.

Studies show that fewer than half of all prescriptions are taken according to the directions on the label. Some patients skip a dose now and then, or they take it at the wrong time. Others go off a medication when they think they don't need it anymore. In one recent study, 85 percent of patients who had been prescribed a heart drug were no longer taking it after two years. Other research shows that some people never even fill their prescription.

The problem of noncompliance—failing to follow doctors' orders—costs thousands of lives a year. Case in point: the latest generation of cholesterol-lowering drugs. Experts say that these pills could save tens of thousands of lives in the United States annually. Yet in a study of individuals given prescriptions for one of these drugs, only one in five patients was still taking the pills as directed after a year.

Noncompliance is one reason a shocking 82 percent of people with coronary artery disease—those at high risk of a heart attack—still have cholesterol levels in the danger zone. Even many heart attack survivors fail to take clot-dissolving medications as directed, drastically increasing their risk of a second heart attack.

The news is no better on the high blood pressure front. One in four Americans has hypertension. Yet only about three in five are even aware that they have the condition, and fewer are being treated for it. According to a recent study, only 17 percent of people who know they have hypertension have it under control.

Excuses, excuses, excuses

Why do so many of us ignore our doctors' orders? Researchers who study the problem of noncompliance have heard every excuse in the book from patients they've interviewed. Here are some common ones—along with good reasons not to skip those pills.

"I didn't think I needed the medication any longer." When a drug makes you better, it makes sense to think you don't need it any longer, right? Wrong. Drugs to control blood pressure or cholesterol typically have to be taken for years, even for the rest of your life. In a recent Scandinavian study, 30 percent of patients who stopped taking cholesterol-lowering drugs said they did so because their cholesterol levels

Key Finding

Want to live longer? Take your cholesterol-lowering medicine. According to findings from the West of Scotland Coronary Prevention Study, patients who took 75 percent or more of the recommended doses of a cholesterol-lowering drug cut their risk of premature death by one-third more than those patients who took less than 75 percent of the pills they had been prescribed.

were now "normal." When the drugs are stopped, unfortunately, cholesterol levels often climb back up.

"I was never really convinced the medicine worked in the first place." To take a drug regularly, every day or even several times a day, you've got to be convinced that it's doing you some good. If you're not sure you really need the medicine your doctor has prescribed, say so right away. Explain your doubts. Ask your doctor what the medicine is supposed to do and what evidence there is that it works. The more you know about the benefits and side effects of a drug, the more likely you are to stick to the regimen.

"I'm worried about the side effects." Many of the newest heart disease drugs have fewer and less serious side effects than earlier ones. Still, potent drugs often have some side effects. Talk to your doctor about what to expect. If you notice symptoms that worry you after you start on a drug, call your doctor immediately. In some cases, side effects go away as your body gets used to the medication. If they don't, your doctor may be able to switch you to a different drug.

"I have trouble remembering to take a drug more than once a day." You're not alone. Studies show that compliance falls off steeply when patients are asked to take a drug more than once a day. That's not surprising. It's simple enough to remember to swallow your pills every morning. But if you have to take one at noon and another in the evening, it's easy to get distracted and forget. If that sounds like you, ask your doctor if another drug is available that can be taken only once a day. Otherwise, turn the page for some ways to help you stick to your regimen.

"I'm worried about the cost." Sadly, this is one of the leading reasons that people go off their medications. Drug costs are high, and many insurance plans cover only part of the price. If money is a concern, talk to your doctor. He or she may be able to prescribe a cheaper drug or at least convince you that the benefits of the drug are worth paying for, even if you have to scrimp on other costs.

"I never thought the problem was that big a deal in the first place." This is another one of the top reasons people don't follow their doctors' advice. Of course it's easy to think elevated

TROUBLESHOOTING

Whenever you fill a prescription, double-check to make sure you're getting the right drug in the right dosage. When researchers analyzed 9,846 prescriptions filled at a large hospital's outpatient pharmacy in New Jersey, they found 1,371 mistakes, ranging from bottles containing the wrong pills or the wrong dosage to labeling errors. In other words, mistakes were made in roughly one in eight of the prescriptions. When in doubt, ask the pharmacist to double-check your prescription.

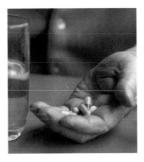

FAST FACT

Failure to follow

medication instructions

is blamed for 10 to 25

percent of all hospital

and nursing home

admissions.

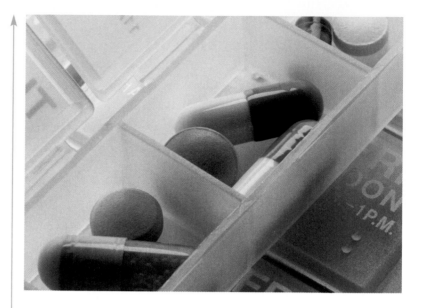

cholesterol or high blood pressure isn't that serious, since neither usually has symptoms. If you're not convinced the problem is worth treating, ask your doctor to explain why he or she thinks it's important to take a medication.

Tips for minding your medicine

Not everyone deliberately skips pills or neglects to refill prescriptions, of course. More often, people just forget. Especially if you have to take a prescribed drug several times during the day—or several medications that have different schedules—it's easy to become confused and miss a dose. Or two. Studies have shown that the more drugs people are taking, the more likely they are to run into trouble following directions. If that sounds like you, these simple tips can help.

- Take your one-a-day medications at the same time every day so you'll be less likely to forget. (Check with your doctor to make sure it's okay.)
- Time your pill-taking with something else that's part of your everyday routine—brushing your teeth, for instance, or eating breakfast (as long as you can take your pills with food).
- Use a pill organizer, available at most pharmacies. Choose one that you can open and close easily and that contains enough compartments for the various pills you take. Some let you set out a week's worth of pills and even provide different compartments for pills taken at different times of day.

- If you have a personal computer, program it to give you a daily reminder. Most calendar and scheduling programs will buzz or beep or post an on-screen reminder. These are especially useful if you work on your computer or check your e-mail several times a day. Of course, you can always set an old-fashioned clock radio or alarm to remind you when it's time to take your pills. Reset it after it rings if you have to take pills more than once a day.
- Call your answering machine and leave a message reminding you to take your medicine. Don't erase it. That way, every time you check your messages, you'll be reminded.

HIGH-TECH REMINDERS

Some people need more than just a note on the fridge to help them remember to take their medicine. If you're one of them, there are several types of products on the market that can help. Some of these clever devices can be found in drugstores. Others can be ordered online at websites such as www.epill.com or www.eldercarechoices.com. For more information, talk to your doctor or pharmacist.

■ **Automated pillboxes.**
Instead of a container that merely holds your pills, how about one that reminds you to take them? Automated pillboxes are available that vibrate, sound an alarm, or offer spoken reminders when your medications are due. More expensive models automatically dispense pills, opening the appropriate compartment when it's time for your medicine. Cost depends on size and how fancy the system is.

Basic models go for as little as $50; the fanciest as much as $800.

■ **Pocket dispensers.** These handy little containers, which fit in your pocket, carry a day's worth of tablets and beep when it's time to take them. Also available are alarms that attach conveniently to your pill bottle.

■ **Messaging services.** For a monthly fee a messaging service will call you at home or on your cell phone when it's time to take your medicine. Alternatively, the service can beep your pager. The cost varies depending on how many calls a day you'll need and the distance of the call. Messaging services can also notify your pharmacist or physician when your medication is running low.

■ **Watches.** Specially designed watches not only tell the time but also beep, flash, or vibrate when it's time for your medicine. Some even display the name of the pill to take.

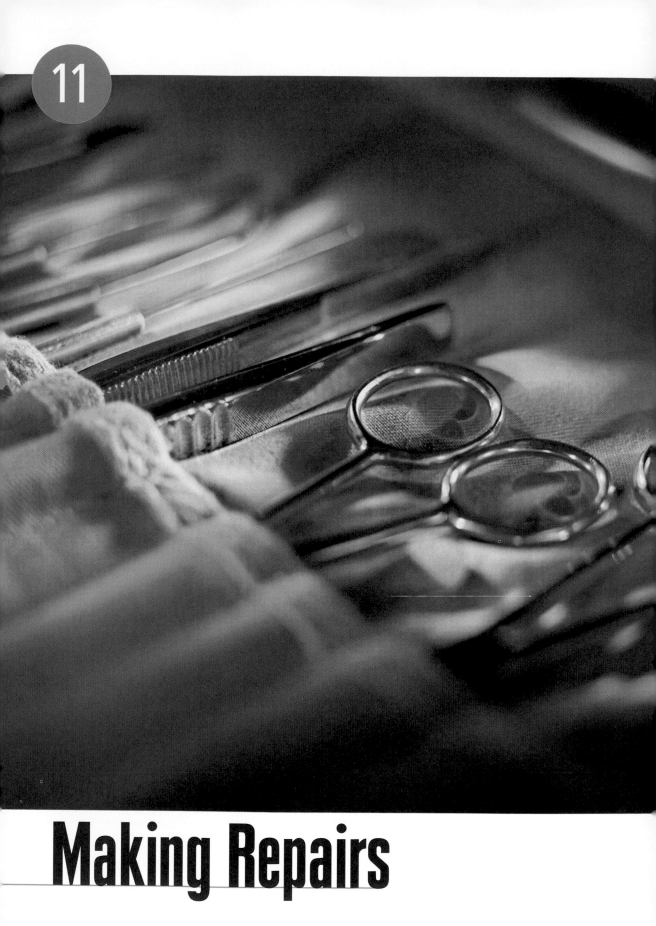

11

Making Repairs

Headlines in 2001 trumpeted a genuine medical miracle: the implanting of the first self-contained mechanical heart inside the chest of a desperately ill man. Although less heralded, many other advances in the field of cardiac surgery have made it possible for surgeons to mend damaged hearts and unclog blocked arteries—bringing new hope to hundreds of thousands of heart patients every year.

It's now routine for surgeons to take blood vessels from one part of the body and reconnect them near the heart to bypass blocked coronary arteries. Even heart transplants, once revolutionary, have become commonplace, with more than 2,500 such surgeries performed in the United States annually. Still more amazing possibilities lie ahead. Researchers are testing a technique that uses light energy to melt away plaque in congested arteries, for instance. And there's exciting evidence that it may be possible to grow new heart muscle to replace tissue damaged during a heart attack. Eventually, researchers say, they may have the means to grow a whole new heart.

The most important advances—at least in terms of lives saved—have been in the treatment of blocked arteries. While medications that widen blood vessels and take the burden off the heart can go a long way toward relieving the symptoms of coronary artery disease, for many patients drugs aren't enough. When arteries become so obstructed that the risk of a heart attack shoots into the red zone, doctors turn to coronary bypass surgery or angioplasty. High-tech innovations are making both options safer and more effective than ever before. And new approaches, such as gene therapy, may one day make both of them obsolete.

High-tech innovations are making angioplasty and coronary bypass surgery safer and more effective than ever before.

Coronary Bypass Surgery

When bypass surgery was first performed more than 25 years ago, it must have seemed as miraculous as the implanting of an artificial heart does today. Coronary artery bypass grafting, as the procedure is technically known, begins with the removal of a blood vessel from a patient's leg, chest, elbow, or stomach. The vessel is then reconnected near the heart in order to bypass a clogged coro-

HOT TOPIC
To Stop or Not to Stop the Heart?

Increasingly, doctors are performing bypass operations "off pump." Instead of using a heart-lung machine, or pump, to stop the heart, they operate while the heart is still beating. First, medications are used to slow the heart rate way down. Then special clamps are used to hold blood vessels still, even while blood is moving through, allowing surgeons to operate on them. In some cases, blood flow can be shut off briefly to specific blood vessels.

Some surgeons prefer off-pump bypass surgery because they believe it lowers the risks associated with stopping a patient's heart and using a heart-lung machine. (There's some evidence that being on a heart-lung machine can cause the loss of a small number of brain cells, although most doctors say the danger is minimal.) But the procedure remains controversial. Critics worry that the advantages of off-pump surgery are outweighed by the fact that surgeons have to work faster and, because the heart is still beating, don't have as much flexibility to move vessels and manipulate the heart in order to reach obstructed arteries. Especially when several bypasses must be performed, they say, the traditional bypass is still the best bet.

nary artery, creating a new channel for blood flow to the heart. When more than one vessel is obstructed, multiple grafts can be attached. Recently, surgeons have also had success rerouting an artery that normally supplies the chest with blood so that it feeds the heart instead.

The vessels that surgeons use for grafting are veins that aren't essential to normal blood flow—hence they can be removed and rerouted without causing blood loss elsewhere. (One commonly used vessel is the saphenous vein, in the leg, which is the same one that is sometimes stripped out to treat varicose veins.) Why use a patient's own blood vessel and not a transplant or an artificial one? First, because the body won't reject it, as it would a transplanted blood vessel. Living vessels can also respond to blood flow by expanding or contracting as necessary—something artificial vessels couldn't do.

A quarter century after it was first pioneered, coronary artery bypass grafting is still widely performed today. And thanks to many refinements over the years, this remarkable surgery now boasts a 98 percent success rate. That's not bad for an operation that requires surgeons to open up the chest by splitting the sternum (breastbone) down the middle, shut down the heart and turn its function over to a heart-lung machine, and then rearrange the circulatory system's plumbing.

Bypass surgery isn't a cure for heart disease, although it does help patients with severe coronary artery disease stay alive. By allowing more blood to reach the heart, it cuts the risk of heart attack in half. It is also remarkably effective for easing severe angina. Eighty percent of patients who undergo the procedure remain free of the crushing chest pain associated with coronary artery disease for at least five years.

Better bypasses

Researchers continue to devise ingenious ways to make bypass surgery even safer and more effective. One involves how surgeons connect grafted blood vessels. Traditionally, they have sewn the vessels into place with sutures. Two new techniques are faster and simpler. One uses stainless-steel clips with tiny hooks that grab onto the artery where the graft is connected. Another uses an adhesive material to connect and seal blood vessels.

Speed is the key advantage. A skilled surgeon can take up to seven minutes to stitch one end of a vessel into place. The suture-less techniques require less than two minutes. Saving five minutes may not sound like a lot, but in operations that require many connections, those minutes add up. And the less time patients have to be on heart-lung machines, the less danger to the heart.

Another major advance: the development of less invasive bypass surgeries. In traditional bypasses, surgeons crack the sternum and fold back the rib cage to get to the heart. A new variation, called minimally invasive direct coronary artery bypass, or MIDCAB, allows surgeons access by way of strategically placed incisions. Part of a rib is sometimes removed to provide a window to the heart.

MIDCAB isn't for everyone. Only about 10 percent of bypass patients qualify. The reason: The procedure is most effective when used to bypass

Heart Doctors Typically Turn to Surgery When:

✔ Patients experience angina even when sitting still

✔ Drugs aren't enough to ease angina

✔ Angina attacks last 20 minutes or more

✔ The risk of a heart attack is high

✔ Arteries are almost completely blocked

✔ More than three coronary arteries are affected

Key Finding

Being sick can make almost anyone feel down. But undergoing heart bypass surgery may be particularly hard on your mental health, doctors are discovering. In one recent study, 65 percent of bypass patients were depressed three weeks after surgery. Twenty-six percent remained depressed 12 weeks later. Researchers speculate that the unique nature of traditional bypass operations, which require stopping the heart and putting patients on heart-lung machines, may be more traumatic emotionally than other kinds of surgery. Researchers are just beginning to look into ways to ease the depression that often follows bypass surgery. The best antidote, many suspect, is to encourage patients to become physically active as soon as possible after the operation.

IS SURGERY REALLY NECESSARY?

Surprisingly, choosing between medication and surgery isn't always easy. Thanks to recent advances, both approaches are yielding better outcomes. For some patients, in fact, they may be equally effective.

Researchers at the University of Washington analyzed results from more than a dozen separate clinical trials involving thousands of patients treated for coronary artery disease. They found that 90 percent of patients given drugs to help keep blood flowing to their hearts were still alive five years later compared with 94 percent of patients who underwent heart bypass surgery. Bypasses were initially more effective at relieving angina. But after five years, the patients on drug therapy experienced just as much relief.

In some cases drugs are actually more effective than surgery. In 1999 *The New England Journal of Medicine* reported surprising results from a study of 341 patients with coronary artery disease who were experiencing only mild to moderate angina. Half were randomly assigned to receive a cholesterol-lowering drug; the others underwent angioplasty. Eighteen months later only 22 percent of those taking the medication had experienced chest pain compared with 37 percent of the angioplasty patients.

How do doctors decide which path to take? The severity of symptoms is one factor. If you have unstable angina—chest pain that occurs even when you aren't exerting yourself—or your angina attacks last for 20 minutes or more, you may be a candidate for surgery. And if you've been on medications, but they aren't doing enough to relieve angina, surgery may be the next step. The extent of the blockages in your coronary arteries is another consideration. And if more than two coronary arteries are blocked, doctors usually opt for surgery.

Another deciding factor is age. Surprisingly, patients aged 75 or older seem to fare better with bypass surgery than medication. In one recent study half of those on medication had experienced a heart attack or other coronary event compared with only 19 percent of those who had received bypasses or angioplasties.

Of course the choice isn't always one or the other. Many doctors use both in an effort to bypass or remove coronary artery obstructions and ensure that they don't recur.

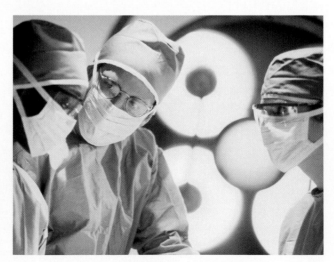

clogged arteries at the front of the heart, which are readily accessible through a small incision. If several arteries are blocked, surgeons typically turn to traditional bypass.

Growing new blood vessels

Researchers may soon have a bold new way to give traditional bypasses a boost. In research funded by the National Heart, Lung, and Blood Institute, Harvard scientists inserted timed-release capsules containing a substance that promotes the growth of new blood vessels into the heart muscle of patients scheduled for bypass surgery. A second group of patients were given a placebo substance. Tests showed that those who received the active substance, called basic fibroblast growth factor, had better blood flow into their heart muscles than those who were given the placebo. They were also less likely to suffer angina after surgery. By spurring the growth of small blood vessels, researchers believe, growth factors ensure that blood from the grafted artery reaches more parts of the heart.

Indeed, growth factors like these may eventually offer an alternative to surgery. In 2001 researchers injected the gene for a growth-promoting substance called vascular endothelial growth factor, or VEGF, directly into the hearts of patients with advanced coronary artery disease who were too sick to undergo surgery. The gene stimulates the production of a naturally occurring protein involved in growing new blood vessels. In one study using VEGF, a majority of patients reported less angina and greater mobility after the treatment. In another study involving 30 patients, 27 reported fewer angina attacks and said they took less nitroglycerin after the treatment.

For now VEGF remains experimental. But if studies underway confirm its effectiveness and safety, it could become one of the first approved uses of gene therapy to treat heart disease.

A Is for Angioplasty

In recent years cardiologists have increasingly turned to a less invasive way to resupply blood to the heart: a technique called percutaneous transluminal coronary angioplasty, or angioplasty for short. Instead of bypassing blocked coronary arteries, doctors reopen obstructed vessels, allowing more blood to flow through them. Angioplasty is especially useful for relieving angina.

FAST FACT

Doctors perform about 300,000 coronary bypass operations every year in the United States.

The procedure involves threading a flexible tube called a catheter, about the diameter of a pencil, through a small incision, usually made in the groin or the arm, and into a main artery. The catheter is then guided into the coronary arteries. Radioactive dye is injected in order to create an X-ray image of the area around the heart. Surgeons use this picture to find the exact location of the obstruction. Then they can clear away the blockage and reopen the clogged blood vessel. The most common technique used to do this, called balloon angioplasty, employs a catheter that has a tiny balloon attached to its tip. Once the tip reaches the obstruction, the balloon is inflated and deflated several times, compressing the fatty deposits in the artery against the vessel wall and thereby reopening the channel. Another, less common technique, called an atherectomy, employs a catheter tipped with a miniature cutting tool, something like a dentist's drill, to file away the cholesterol-laden plug blocking blood flow.

Risks and benefits

By allowing more blood to reach the heart, angioplasty dramatically reduces symptoms of angina and cuts the risk of a heart attack. But there's a catch: The procedure itself can sometimes trigger a heart attack. As cholesterol-laden plaque is broken down during the operation, tiny pieces may break loose and flow downstream into smaller arteries, creating a jam, known as an embolism, and blocking blood flow.

The risk of a heart attack triggered by angioplasty is generally about 5 percent. But the danger can jump as high as 15 percent in patients who have bypass grafts or stents in place. The good news: Clever gadgets called embolization protection devices promise to lower the risk dramat-

Key Finding

Folic acid, a B vitamin, has long been known to lower homocysteine levels, which in turn is associated with reduced heart disease risk. Now a new finding published in the November 2001 *New England Journal of Medicine* shows that folic acid can also ward off restenosis. In a study of 205 angioplasty patients, half were given a folic-acid supplement, the rest a placebo pill. Six months later those on the folic-acid therapy had lower levels of homocysteine in their blood—and their blood was much more likely to be flowing freely. The rate of restenosis was only 20 percent in the folic-acid group compared with 38 percent in the placebo group.

REAL PEOPLE, REAL WISDOM

Get Moving to Get Well

"I stand before you a man with nine bypasses," says Jack French, 64. "I can tell you right now, I'm doing just fine. And I plan to go on doing just fine."

French was just 42, working as a salesman who traveled a five-state territory around Alabama, when he had his first bypass operation. "I was walking into a shopping mall in Columbus, Georgia, with my sample case when it hit me—a pain like a truck slamming into my chest," he recalls. When doctors found major blockages in several of his arteries, they rushed him into surgery.

"That first operation, they did six separate bypasses on me. I was in the hospital for three days. A week after, I was raking leaves in the backyard. And it wasn't long before I was back to work," he remembers. He was also back to his old ways of eating, swilling down half a dozen Cokes a day and eating buckets of fried chicken. At 5 feet 10 inches, he weighed 280 pounds.

Eventually, those habits caught up with him again. When French decided to retire, he scheduled a physical exam. Doctors discovered that the grafted arteries had developed new blockages—and French underwent a second operation, this one involving three grafts.

"The second time I was in the hospital just two days, and when I got out I figured I'd just bounce back, like I had the first time," he recalls. But it wasn't that easy. He found himself feeling isolated and depressed. "That's something the doctors don't tell you about, the depression. You can find yourself getting so anxious you're afraid of doing anything for fear of doing more damage to your heart."

Luckily for him, the heart clinic at the University of Alabama at Birmingham offered a six-week cardiac rehabilitation program that helped him get back on his feet. Luckily, too, the doctors convinced him it was time to make some big changes in his diet.

Today, the man who used to eat a big steak almost every other day now limits himself to a small T-bone once a week. Instead of fried chicken, his favorite dinner is now red snapper. He's given up soft drinks for water. He begins every morning with a bowl of instant oatmeal and eats more fruit daily—oranges, apples, pears, apricots—than he used to eat in a year.

To shake the depression, French took up landscaping—building walls and putting in rock gardens on the two acres he and his wife have in Pelham, just outside Birmingham. Today, two years after his second bypass surgery, he's up at six most mornings and in the garden at eight. And he often doesn't knock off work until five. He's dropped 80 pounds and feels more energetic than he has in a long time. "I tell people that the best way to get well is to get moving," says French. "The doctors can do wonders for you. But you've got to do the rest for yourself."

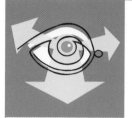

LOOKING AHEAD

Melting plaques with light

Even in the most skilled hands, catheters used during angioplasty can damage artery walls, making the arteries more vulnerable to new blockages. A gentler approach to clearing away coronary artery obstructions could solve the problem. In an experimental technique called photoangioplasty, surgeons use infrared light to melt away plaques without touching healthy artery cells around them. First, they inject a light-sensitive chemical that is absorbed by the plaque but not the surrounding cells. Then a very narrow catheter is guided to the site, where it emits high-frequency light energy. This energy stimulates the light-sensitive chemical, which in turn destroys the obstruction, leaving healthy cells undisturbed. Although photoangioplasty is still in the early stages of testing, many researchers think it will offer an effective alternative to standard angioplasty in coming years.

ically. The new devices are really nothing more than tiny filters, about the size of a pencil eraser. They are threaded into position downstream of the artery blockage. There, they catch up to 93 percent of the debris that breaks loose.

Another serious problem associated with angioplasties hasn't been as easy to solve. In one out of three patients, blockages re-form in coronary arteries within three to six months after the procedure, a phenomenon called restenosis. The new blockages aren't the same as the cholesterol-laden plaques that cause coronary artery disease in the first place. Small blood clots and cholesterol buildup may play a role; but the real culprit, scientists now think, is damage inflicted on the lining of blood vessels during angioplasty. When the lining is disturbed, immune cells rush in to repair the damage, triggering the growth of new cells. These new cells form thickened patches, a bit like scabs, which in turn reduce blood flow through the artery.

Exactly why some patients suffer restenosis and other don't is still something of a mystery. In a study reported in 2001, researchers from New Zealand followed 2,690 angioplasty patients. Six months after surgery, angiograms showed that 607 of them had developed new blockages. Half of them had no angina symptoms to alert doctors to the problem. Men were more likely than women to have so-called "silent" restenosis. But the researchers found nothing else in the patients' medical histories that would predict who developed restenosis.

When new blockages form, surgeons often have to perform another angioplasty. If blockages recur, bypass surgery may be necessary. Now, however, there's exciting evidence that scientists may have finally put the problem of reblockage to rest.

Block that blockage

The first giant step in preventing restenosis came with the introduction of devices called stents, expandable metal-mesh tubes implanted after an artery is widened in order to keep the channel open. Stents are now implanted in more than two-thirds of all angioplasty patients. These simple devices have proved so successful that more and more surgeons are skipping the balloon entirely and simply using a stent to open clogged arteries. Researchers at the State University of New York at Stony Brook recently reported that this "direct stenting" is just as effective as implanting a stent after balloon angioplasty. And it offers two distinct advantages: shorter operating time and lower costs.

The use of stents has cut the danger of new blockages from about 40 percent to only 15 to 20 percent. And another approach, called coronary brachytherapy, is lowering the risk even further. Surgeons zap the lining of newly unclogged arteries with a small dose of radiation, which has been shown to reduce the occurrence of new obstructions by approximately 60 percent.

Yet another innovation may be even more successful at preventing restenosis. Researchers are testing stents coated with

FAST FACT

More than one million

angioplasties are

performed each year in

the United States.

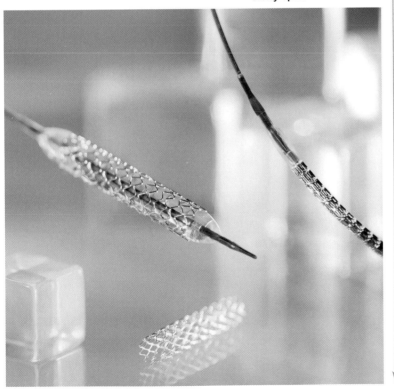

After angioplasty, a small metal tube called a stent may be inserted to keep the artery open.

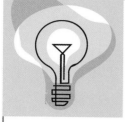

ASK THE EXPERT

With advances coming along so quickly, how can I make sure my doctor is taking advantage of the latest breakthroughs?

Stanley Rockson, M.D., associate professor of cardiovascular medicine at Stanford University:

"It's easy to get caught up in all the excitement surrounding the state-of-the-art techniques making headlines. But it's important to put these new discoveries in perspective. One of the great strengths of our medical system is the push to innovate—to find new and better ways to treat illnesses and help people stay well. But another strength is caution. We insist that new drugs or surgical techniques be carefully tested and the results documented so doctors know what works and what doesn't.

And believe me, there are plenty of examples of promising new ideas that didn't pan out quite the way we expected them to. Take laser angioplasty, for instance. For a time, all of us in the field were very excited about the prospect of using lasers to burn away plaque on the inside of arteries. Mostly we hoped the technique would help prevent restenosis. Hospitals around the country bought hundreds of fancy laser-based angioplasty devices. Unfortunately, laser angioplasty didn't turn out to be any better than the traditional approach, and many of those devices now sit in hospital corridors covered with sheets. Right now there is interest in another new approach, called photoangioplasty, which uses a light-sensitive chemical and infrared light to remove plaque. Only time, and thorough testing, will tell if it is a bona fide advance.

Indeed, it takes three to five years to test a new approach to find out whether it's truly safe and effective—and once something is approved, it takes another three to five years for physicians using it in their practices to decide whether it really is any better than traditional approaches.

For 95 percent or more of patients with coronary artery disease, the best chance of success is tried-and-true treatments with proven value. Certainly if you've read about something that sounds exciting, ask your doctor. But remember, you're usually better off in the hands of a surgeon who is using a technique he or she trusts and has done many times before than with some new and unproven approach."

substances that block excess cell growth. One version is laced with an antibiotic called sirolimus, which prevents cells from multiplying. In results announced in September 2001, researchers reported that seven months after angioplasty, no new blockages had occurred in any of 700 patients given the drug-coated stents.

Which surgery to choose?

How do doctors decide when to perform bypass surgery and when to use angioplasty? The decision typically involves weighing many factors. One important advantage of angioplasty is the fact that it is far less invasive. But it usually isn't as effective in resupplying blood to the heart, especially over the long haul. So doctors often perform angioplasty first, hoping that it will do the trick. If it doesn't, they may turn to bypass surgery.

Sometimes angioplasties aren't practical, however—if too many arteries are blocked, for example, or one artery is obstructed with a blockage so large that the artery can't be opened by a catheter. Surgeons also avoid angioplasty in patients with diabetes. Because the disease causes damage to blood vessels, they worry that the trauma of inserting a catheter could cause further injury. Bypass surgery is a safer bet.

Of course bypasses aren't always practical—when patients are too frail to withstand the operation, for instance. Or when previous bypasses have been performed, and there are no more blood vessels left to graft.

New Approaches, New Hope

When drugs aren't powerful enough, and bypasses or angioplasties aren't practical, there's still hope. Doctors have been experimenting with a technique called transmyocardial revascularization, or TMR, which involves drilling tiny holes into heart muscle. No one really knows why the technique works, although the holes do seem to allow more blood to reach heart muscle cells. Several studies have shown that TMR can bring relief to people with angina. Because the holes eventually heal over, however, the benefits are usually short-lived.

Surprisingly successful for many patients is a technique imported from China called enhanced external counterpulsation, or EECP. To look at it, you wouldn't think EECP had anything to do with the heart. Pressurized cuffs are placed around a patient's upper and lower legs. Then an air pump inflates and deflates the cuffs, squeezing leg muscles and forcing blood up into the heart. The pump is precisely synchronized to inflate the cuffs each time the heart relaxes between beats, producing a "counterpulse" that creates additional blood pressure when blood is refilling the heart's chambers.

Questions to Ask When You Consider Surgery

✔ How is the operation done?

✔ What is the purpose of the operation?

✔ Are there alternatives to surgery?

✔ What will you gain by having the operation?

✔ What are the possible complications and side effects?

✔ Why should the operation be done now?

✔ How often has the surgeon performed this operation?

✔ What is the surgeon's success rate?

✔ What complications has he or she encountered?

✔ How will you feel after the surgery?

✔ How long will your recovery take?

✔ Is there anything you can do to speed your recovery?

Again, scientists aren't exactly sure why counterpulsation seems to ease angina. The technique has been shown to widen arteries that feed the heart, especially smaller arteries that don't normally play a big role in supplying blood to heart muscles. EECP also appears to spur the growth of new coronary arteries. Whatever the mechanism, it seems to work. In a study at the State University of New York at Stony Brook, researchers tested EECP in 18 patients with advanced coronary artery disease. The hour-long procedure was repeated 35 times over 7 weeks. All 18 patients reported significantly less angina. Sixteen were completely free of chest pain during their normal activities. Imaging tests showed that artery blockages were reduced in 14 out of the 18 patients.

For now, doctors perform EECP only when other, more traditional approaches fail. Yet some researchers think that the technique should play a role in treating patients newly diagnosed with coronary artery disease. By stimulating increased blood flow to the heart, EECP could help prevent angina and ward off heart attacks, they say. The problem: Most insurance companies cover the cost of EECP only as a last-ditch measure.

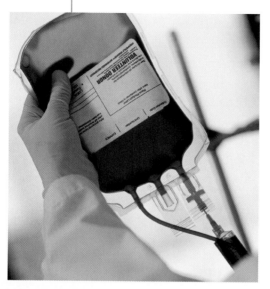

Key Finding

For patients with heart failure, a simple blood transfusion can make a big difference in the odds of survival, according to a 2001 Yale University study. Examining records from 78,974 elderly people, researchers found that 40 percent were anemic. Those with the lowest red blood cell counts were twice as likely as those with normal blood readings to die during the first month after a heart attack. What makes this finding especially worrisome is that only one-quarter of the anemic patients studied were given blood transfusions to boost their red blood cell levels. Patients who did receive transfusions dramatically improved their odds of surviving a heart attack. By publishing their results, the Yale team hopes to encourage doctors to test more patients for anemia—and to offer those with low red blood cell counts potentially lifesaving transfusions.

New Help for Failing Hearts

Coronary artery disease, severe high blood pressure, heart attacks—all three can leave the heart too weak to supply

ASK THE EXPERT

Is it normal to feel anxious or depressed after heart surgery—and is there anything I can do?

John F. Todaro, Ph.D., assistant professor of psychiatry at the Brown Medical School and staff psychologist at Miriam Hospital in Rhode Island:

"Absolutely. Many people who've had a heart attack or undergone cardiac surgery feel anxious or depressed afterward. The experience can be very scary. It's natural to wonder if your heart is going to keep working as it did and whether you'll be able to make the lifestyle changes needed to keep you healthy.

Being alert to how you feel is critical to your recovery. Dozens of studies have shown that anxiety or depression can get in the way of getting well. Stress puts a strain on your heart, increases blood pressure, and can even affect cholesterol levels.

What to look out for? Stress usually shows up in three different ways. There are physiological symptoms, such as muscle tension, racing heart, excess sweating, trembling, and stomach complaints. There are also behavioral symptoms. You may not be sleeping as well as usual. You may suddenly stop getting pleasure out of things you used to love. Or you may notice yourself getting unusually frustrated at the smallest things. Finally, there are cognitive changes—memory loss, poor concentration, and mental confusion.

In our cardiac rehabilitation program, we focus on four main strategies to help heart patients relieve stress and ease depression. The first is learning relaxation techniques—deep-breathing exercises that help people focus their thoughts and relax their muscles. The second strategy is exercise. Physical activities like walking are a great way to manage stress and also get the added heart benefits of exercise.

Third, we encourage people to try to connect with friends and family. Studies show that people who are isolated are more likely to get sick and die than people with a strong social network. So if you belong to a church, now is the time to get more involved. Look for social activities in your community. Or simply call up some old friends and catch up.

Finally, it's important to do things you enjoy. That may sound like common sense. But when people are feeling depressed, they tend to become reclusive. On the other hand, when people pursue pleasurable activities—when they push themselves to get out and go for a walk in a favorite park or see a play or attend a concert— they are able to get themselves out of a rut and feeling better about their lives.

There's another benefit to getting up and doing something. The more you do, the more confident you'll feel about your health. That confidence will help you stay motivated to make the changes necessary to live a heart healthy lifestyle."

enough blood to meet the body's needs. An estimated five million Americans suffer from heart failure. Half a million more are diagnosed each year. Heart medications have made a big difference for many of them. But drugs aren't always powerful enough to ease the burden on failing hearts, and doctors have to turn to surgery.

The little pump that could

At heart, the human heart is a pump—nothing more and nothing less. When hearts fail, the problem usually lies with the left ventricle, the chamber that pumps blood to the entire body. Miniaturized pumps, called ventricular assist devices, can be implanted in the chest to help push blood forward. The newest versions work like tiny jet engines, moving blood at a steady pace.

KEEPING THE PACE

In as many as half the people with heart failure, the left and right ventricles, the heart's main pumping chambers, don't contract at exactly the same time. Blood sloshes back and forth between the chambers rather than being squeezed out to the rest of the body. A new type of pacemaker approved by the FDA in 2001 synchronizes the two chambers, boosting the heart's pumping power and improving the quality of life of the people who receive it. The device allows patients to be more active, less out of breath, and less fatigued.

Pacemakers are small implantable devices that deliver electrical charges to keep the heart beating regularly. Most are used to treat heartbeat irregularities, or arrhythmias. Traditional pacemakers commonly supply two wires to the heart: one to the upper right chamber (the right atrium) and one to the lower right chamber (the right ventricle). The InSync Biventricular Cardiac Pacing System has a third wire that connects to the lower left chamber, synchronizing the two ventricles. Like other high-tech pacemakers, the InSync even slows down or speeds up depending on the person's activity level.

To test the InSync device, researchers implanted the pacemaker (about the size of a quarter) in 532 patients with heart failure but only turned it on in 263 of them. During the next three to six months, the people with the activated pacemaker were able to walk farther and scored higher on a test that measures quality of life. At the end of the study, the researchers turned on the pacemakers in the other patients so that they could benefit from it too.

204

As a result, patients no longer have a normal heartbeat. This lack of a pulse makes it difficult for doctors to measure a patient's blood pressure, since blood pressure gauges depend on counting heartbeats. But even this problem is being solved. The latest pumps can check on conditions in the body and transmit data to physicians to help them monitor their patients.

Traditionally, mechanical pumps have been thought of as a "bridge" treatment—a way to keep patients with serious heart failure alive while they waited for heart transplants. Because donor hearts are so scarce, however, many patients have ended up on these pumps for extended periods of time—in some cases up to four years. Not long ago, researchers began to wonder whether the pumps themselves might offer a permanent alternative to heart transplantation.

Pumps like the HeartMate can help people with serious heart failure live longer.

To find out how well the pumps performed, researchers at the Columbia University College of Physicians and Surgeons in Manhattan enlisted 129 patients with heart failure who were ineligible for transplants because they were either too sick or too old. Some of the volunteers were then given a mechanical pump called the HeartMate, which is implanted in the abdomen. The rest of the volunteers were treated with drugs shown to help ease the burden on failing hearts.

The HeartMate uses one tube to drain blood from the left ventricle into the mechanical pump. Another tube pumps it back into the aorta, from which it flows out to the body. A third passes through the skin to an external battery pack and control system. Nothing fancy, really, but the Columbia study proved that these little pumps are lifesavers. A year after they were installed 52 percent of patients were still alive—compared with only 25 percent of those who received the best available drug treatments. After two years 23 percent of patients with the pumps were still alive compared with only 8 percent of those on medications.

EMERGENCY HELP WHEN YOU NEED IT

An estimated 250,000 Americans die each year of cardiac arrest when their hearts suddenly stop pumping blood. Cardiac arrest is often caused by ventricular fibrillation, when the lower chambers of the heart rapidly contract out of sync. A defibrillator—a device that delivers a jolt of electricity to shock the heart back into beating normally—can save many of those lives, but only if one happens to be available. Too often it isn't. But now the FDA has approved a new defibrillator for patients with severe heart arrhythmias—one that can be worn on the body.

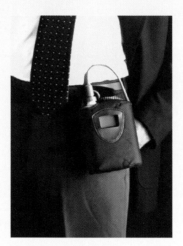

The device, Lifecor's WCD 2000 System, contains four sensors, strapped to the chest, that monitor heartbeat. When they notice an irregular heart rhythm, they signal a miniature defibrillator, worn on a belt around the waist, to deliver a shock to the heart. In a study of 289 patients the device was successful 71 percent of the time in detecting and treating sudden cardiac arrest compared with a success rate of only 25 percent when people call 911. Experts say the device will be useful for people following a serious heart attack and for patients awaiting a heart transplant.

Researchers say mechanical pumps could prevent some 100,000 deaths from heart failure every year. But the price tag is substantial. The cost of installing a pump and monitoring patients runs about $160,000 a year.

The gift of life

The very idea of transplanting a living heart from one person to another still seems miraculous. Yet today some 2,500 heart transplants are performed in the United States each year. Researchers have made giant strides in controlling the biggest problem of transplantation: organ rejection. New drugs effectively suppress the body's immune system so it won't attack the new organ, allowing the transplanted heart to go on beating.

The biggest limitation is a lack of donor hearts. Experts estimate that as many as 50,000 Americans suffering from heart failure need a new heart. Yet there are only about 7,000 potential donors each year. Efforts are underway to improve the organ donor information network so that more hearts and other organs become available. Still, the transplantation of living hearts will never offer a complete solution to the problem of heart failure. As an alternative, researchers have dreamed for years of creating a mechanical organ that would beat as reliably as our own heart. Recently that dream became reality.

The bionic heart comes of age

In July 2001 the world's first truly bionic heart began beating—or rather clicking—in the chest of a human patient. The man who made medical history was a retired telephone company employee named Robert Tools, whose own heart was failing rapidly. As he told reporters at Jewish Hospital in Louisville, Kentucky, where the operation was performed: "I had a choice to sit at home and die or come in here and take a chance."

That chance paid off. The three-pound artificial heart implanted in his chest is nothing short of an engineering marvel. In the past, artificial hearts had to be connected by wires that passed through the skin to a power supply unit, creating a constant risk of serious infection. The newest artificial ticker, called the AbioCor, is equipped with its own rechargeable battery that allows the device to be fully self-contained. Most of the time, a small battery pack worn outside the body sends radio waves to power the AbioCor. But the artificial heart's rechargeable battery can run on its own for up to 45 minutes, allowing patients to bathe or go swimming, for instance. A microchip in the heart allows it to adjust its rate to what patients are doing.

The bionic heart kept Robert Tools alive for 151 days. That may not sound like much. But without it, doctors say, he wouldn't have lived more than a month. To date, almost a dozen patients have received AbioCor hearts. Since the devices are still experimental, only the sickest patients—those for whom all other measures have failed—are candidates to

The AbioCor is the first artificial heart to be fully enclosed inside the body.

207

receive them. In the future, as researchers learn more about how these mechanical wonders perform, they expect to be able to treat individuals with less advanced heart failure—and a better chance of long-term survival.

More Wonders Ahead

It's remarkable enough that surgeons have learned how to transplant living hearts and construct an entirely artificial one. But what if researchers could somehow discover a way to encourage damaged hearts to heal themselves? What if they could trigger the body to grow new heart muscle—or even a whole new heart?

Such hopes were the stuff of science fiction until recently. Now several studies offer stunning evidence that heart muscle can be regenerated and, possibly, new hearts grown.

Researchers have known for years that the bone marrow, the liver, and the lining of the intestines can regenerate, replacing damaged or diseased tissue with new healthy cells. But most experts assumed that the heart lacked the ability to grow new cells. Then, in 2001, investigators from New York Medical College discovered something startling: what looked like brand-new heart muscle cells in areas near where a heart attack had occurred. At the time, the scientists didn't know whether these were simply existing heart cells that had divided to form new cells or entirely new cells, born of stem cells, the progenitors of all the body's specialized tissues.

Now they know, thanks to a clever experiment reported in *The*

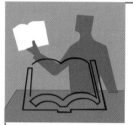

TERMS TO KNOW

ANGIOPLASTY A procedure in which a narrow tube called a catheter is threaded into blocked coronary arteries in order to clear an obstruction, often using a tiny balloon that's inflated and deflated several times to reopen the vessel

CORONARY ARTERY BYPASS GRAFTING An operation that involves removing a blood vessel from the leg or other part of the body and grafting it near the heart to bypass a clogged coronary artery

EMBOLISM A blood clot that forms in a blood vessel in one part of the body and travels to another part

PACEMAKER A miniature electronic device implanted in the chest and wired to the heart to control the heartbeat

RESTENOSIS The formation of new blockages after either angioplasty or bypass surgery has been performed

STEM CELLS Primitive cells created in the bone marrow that can develop into any of the many specialized cells of the body

STENT An expandable metal-mesh tube that is placed inside an obstructed artery to widen the vessel and keep it open

New England Journal of Medicine in January 2002. The New York Medical College team transplanted eight hearts from female donors into male patients. When they looked at new heart muscle cells that had arisen, they found that 10 percent of them contained a Y chromosome, the definitive marker of a male cell. The evidence proved that stem cells from the patients had migrated into the heart and were helping to replace muscle cells injured during the transplant operation.

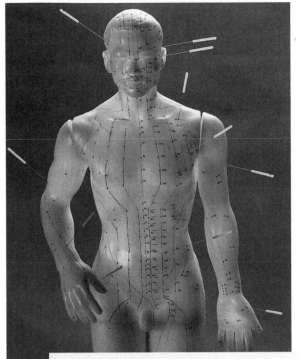

This extraordinary finding raises hopes that scientists may eventually be able to harness the power of stem cells, encouraging the heart to repair itself after a heart attack or other injury. Indeed, some scientists are already trying to do exactly that. In a study reported in 2001, French doctors implanted stem cells from a heart patient's thigh muscle into his ailing heart, in anticipation that the cells would develop into healthy heart muscle cells.

Key Finding

One of the world's oldest healing techniques may help people with severe heart failure, according to results reported at the American Heart Association's 2001 conference. Acupuncture, the practice of inserting needles into the skin at specific points, was shown to ease the burden on ailing hearts by reducing sympathetic nerve activity. (The sympathetic nervous system, or "emergency response system," is charged with increasing heart rate and blood pressure and rushing blood into the muscles as part of the "fight or flight" response.) That's important, because heart failure patients have two to three times more sympathetic nerve activity than healthy people. The greater that activity, the worse the prognosis. Further studies are needed to confirm the new promise of this ancient technique.

Preliminary results suggest the new cells have indeed strengthened the heart. Eventually, experts say, as they learn more about what triggers stem cells to differentiate into specialized tissues, they may be able to grow new hearts for people with heart disease.

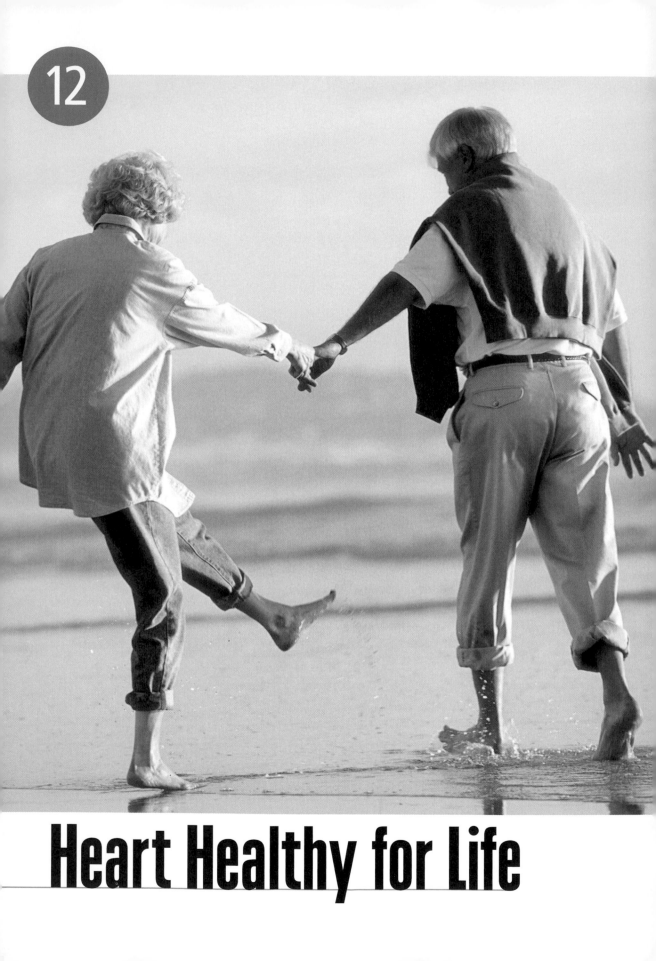

Heart Healthy for Life

There's no doubt about it: Cardiologists today can work wonders for the heart. But the most powerful medicine is still what you do for yourself. That's true even after you've suffered a heart attack or undergone heart surgery. The same steps that can help prevent heart disease in the first place—from eating a smarter diet to injecting more physical activity into your routine—will speed your recovery and dramatically reduce your odds of further trouble.

The fact is, it's never too late to start taking care of your heart. If you're a smoker who's had a heart attack, for instance, you can cut your risk of having another in half by kicking the habit now. If you've been diagnosed with coronary artery disease, lifestyle changes can actually reverse the process of atherosclerosis, opening up clogged arteries. There another benefit: Starting healthy new habits now can help you regain a sense of control over your health and feel more positive about the future.

Lifestyle plays such a powerful role in helping heart patients recover after a heart attack or surgery that many medical centers now offer formal cardiac rehabilitation programs. There's no magic to these programs. Most focus on that familiar threesome: exercise, diet, and stress reduction. The real benefit is the close supervision and encouragement they offer, as well as the support of other patients in the same situation. Several studies have shown that people who enroll in cardiac rehab get better and become active sooner than those who don't.

If a rehab program is available to you, by all means take advantage of it. If not, don't despair. With your doctor's help, you can create your own program for recovery.

On the Road to Recovery

The first thing to focus on is becoming physically active again. There was a time when cardiologists counseled patients to take it easy, even to remain in bed for weeks after a heart attack or surgery. Not any more. The sooner you get up and get moving, experts now say, the faster you'll recover—even if you've had very

If you've been diagnosed with coronary artery disease, lifestyle changes can actually reverse the process of atherosclerosis, opening up clogged arteries.

serious heart problems. If you were a couch potato before, your doctor will probably counsel you to become more active than you were. Otherwise, the goal is to resume your former exercise habits.

How much can you safely do? That's a question for your cardiologist to answer. Most rehab programs encourage people to begin slowly and gradually add more—and more strenuous—activities, beginning with walking and progressing to pedaling on a stationary bike, jogging, swimming, or other activities. How hard you should push yourself depends on what you've just been through, how active you were in the past, and your overall health. Your ultimate goal should be at least 30 minutes of moderately intense exercise—a brisk walk or the equivalent—most days of the week.

Naturally, it's smart to listen to your body. If you experience chest pain while working out, tell your doctor. Discuss any worries you have about physical activity. But don't let fear stop you from reaping the benefits of exercise. Consider this: In a study of 68 patients so sick that they were on a waiting list for heart transplants, an exercise program alone proved so successful at easing their symptoms and improving coronary artery blood flow that 31 were healthy enough to be removed from the transplant list!

Once you're up and moving again, it's time to take a fresh look at your diet. There's nothing new about the advice. Cut back on saturated fat. Consume more fruits and vegetables. Load up on whole-grain foods. But there's new urgency if you've been diagnosed with heart disease. One of the major benefits of a heart-smart diet is its effect on LDL cholesterol, the artery-clogging kind. And if you have coronary artery disease, you need to strive to get your LDL level down even farther than people whose arteries are clear. According to experts from the National Cholesterol Education Program, people with zero or one risk factor can get away with an LDL level under 160 mg/dL. People with two or more risk factors should strive to get theirs below 130 mg/dL. But if you have heart disease, your ideal LDL level is under 100 mg/dL. Your doctor may recommend a cholesterol-lowering drug to bring your numbers down. But everything you do to improve your diet will help.

TROUBLESHOOTING TIP

Men suffering from heart failure often have trouble maintaining erections because their hearts can't pump enough blood throughout the body. Exercise can help, according to a study by experts at the Lancisi Heart Institute in Italy. Among a group of 59 men with heart failure, those who cycled 40 minutes three times a week for eight weeks dramatically improved their scores on a standard questionnaire used to gauge sexual function. They also improved their overall quality of life.

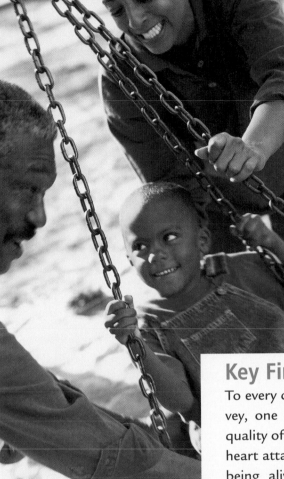

Key Finding

To every cloud there's a silver lining. In a recent survey, one out of three patients reported that their quality of life had actually improved after suffering a heart attack. Patients pointed to an increased joy in being alive, closer relationships with their loved ones, a clearer grasp of what really matters in their lives, and an increased sense of well-being thanks to healthier habits.

Finally, there's the issue of stress. Finding ways to relax is a good idea no matter what your state of health, but it's even more important if you've been diagnosed with heart disease. Any serious illness creates its own stresses. It can even force difficult decisions, such as whether to keep working or retire. Unfortunately, the same emotional strain caused by heart disease can slow your recovery. In fact, a high degree of psychological stress after a heart attack has been shown to be an independent risk factor for dying within the next year.

The good news: Even in the face of something as serious as heart disease, simple relaxation techniques can make a real difference. In one study, researchers compared a group of heart patients who were given relaxation audio tapes in the cardiac care unit with patients who received standard care. The tapes contained spoken instructions for progressive muscle relaxation and deep breathing exercises. Four months later, the patients who received the tapes were walking further and suffering fewer episodes of chest pain. Just as important, half as many as those in the other group reported having emotional difficulties. You can find a variety of relaxation tapes at bookstores and online. Many medical centers offer stress reduction programs that include both counseling and tools such as tapes.

REAL PEOPLE, REAL WISDOM

Life After a Heart Attack

"Oh, I used to talk the talk, all right," Grace Lennox, 67, says with a laugh. "But it wasn't until I had my heart attack that I really began to walk the walk."

It's been almost 10 years since her husband called 911 and she was rushed to the emergency room in St. Louis. "I was lucky. They got to me soon enough, and the attack wasn't so bad that it caused any kind of serious damage. But let me tell you, after that, I decided it was time for a change."

Like many women, Lennox had focused a lot of her energy on her family—her husband and three boys. But after suffering a heart attack, she decided it was high time to start taking better care of herself.

"I knew all that fried food wasn't good for me. I knew I was heavier than I should be. I'd see ladies out there in sweatpants, walking through the neighborhood, and I'd say to myself, 'Honey, you've got to start getting yourself some exercise.' But I guess I never really believed it. Or I just never seemed to

have the time." Once she got out of the hospital, Lennox says, she made the time.

"I remember sitting down and making a list of things I was going to do, right then and there. One of them was to get a low-fat cookbook. Another was to get my own pair of sweatpants and start walking."

In a sense, she recalls, it almost helped to have a serious health emergency pull her up short. "Having that heart attack really made me take a look at myself," says Lennox. "It really made me get my priorities straight. That was my wake-up call, let me tell you. It made me stop and say, hey, wait just a minute. This isn't who I want to be. This isn't the way I want to be living."

Today, 30 pounds lighter and more active than she's ever been in her life, Lennox says she no longer thinks of herself as someone with heart disease. "There was the old me, and there's the new me," she says. And then she laughs again. "Honey, I don't need to tell you which one I like better."

Meeting the Challenge Ahead

Remember the old bumper sticker that read "Today is the first day of the rest of your life"? Sure it's a cliché. But it also captures an essential truth. Today really can be the beginning of a healthier life. New drugs and treatments can help. But the rest is up to you.

No one's saying it will always be easy. Even people who have been called to action by serious heart problems sometimes find it difficult to overcome a lifetime of unhealthy habits. They may be enthusiastic at first—or at least grimly determined. But after the first month, researchers find, people's commitment begins to fade. By the end of six months, evidence shows, too many have abandoned their best intentions.

Why? One reason is almost certainly that, like the proverbial old dog, it's not easy for people to learn new tricks. Habits have a way of becoming deeply ingrained. And it's not just a matter of being stuck in a rut. Some habits, like smoking, are physically addictive. Others become hard-wired into our brains, much the same way a learned skill like riding a bike becomes programmed into our neural pathways. Anything we repeat again and again becomes a learned behavior. That's great, if all your habits are healthy ones. If they're not, breaking them can be a challenge.

But it can be done. If you get into the practice of walking around the neighborhood instead of turning on the tube after dinner, you'll gradually find it's easier to hit the sidewalk instead of the couch. Make a habit of having fruit for dessert, and it won't take long before you're looking forward to the taste of a baked apple, a bowl of ripe cherries, or orange and grapefruit sections splashed with liqueur. You won't erase the old habit. Chances are you'll still be tempted to vegetate in front of the TV after dinner, in other words. And no doubt you'll want to treat yourself to a slice of cheesecake now and then. (And once in a while you should.) But the longer you stick with a new routine, the easier it will be to shun the old temptations.

Become a rebel with a cause

There's another reason that living heart healthy is so tough: the world we live in. Some scientists have gone so far as to describe it as a toxic environment because of how it seduces us to make

> Make a habit of having fruit for dessert, and it won't take long before you're looking forward to the taste.

4 Inspiring Truths About Change

1

"Human beings, by changing the inner attitudes of their minds, can change the outer aspects of their lives." –Psychologist William James

2

"Only I can change my life. No one can do it for me." –Actress Carol Burnett

3

"Always bear in mind that your own resolution to success is more important than any other one thing." –President Abraham Lincoln

4

"Decide what you want, decide what you are willing to exchange for it. Establish your priorities and go to work." –Essayist H.L. Hunt

unhealthy choices. Turn on the television, and you'll be besieged with ads for greasy fast foods and sugary cereals. And everywhere you look, new devices are making life more and more sedentary— from people-movers at airports to on-line shopping. Not long ago, a new invention was unveiled with all kinds of fanfare: a scooter-like device that practically steers itself, allowing people to ride rather than walk down even the most crowded sidewalk. If it catches on, walking may become a thing of the past!

The bottom line is clear: It takes a conscious decision to resist many of the messages being trumpeted around us. The best way to start is to think of yourself as a rebel with a very important cause: your own health and well-being.

Secrets to Success

It's not surprising, especially after you discover you have heart trouble, to want to rush in and change everything at once. And for some people, a crash program of sweeping reforms works just fine. As long as they have to make adjustments, they say, they'd rather do it all at once.

But there may be a hidden danger in this approach. People who charge ahead in a hurry sometimes have trouble maintaining the changes they've made. For starters, their determination may burn out early, before they've had time to turn their new habits into settled ways of living. What's more, they have a tendency to think of change as all or nothing. And when something comes along that knocks them off track—and almost everyone hits a bump in the road now and then—they can quickly become discouraged and give up.

A surer way to make lasting changes, psychologists say, is step by step, making one moderate change, feeling comfortable with it, and then making another. If you've altered your habits gradually, it may be easier to adjust them when times get hard. If you went from three walks a week to four and then five, it's no big deal to downshift to fewer walks when life becomes hectic. And when it eases up, you know what it takes to increase your activities again.

Research in the field of behavioral change has revealed several other strategies that are particularly important to success over the long term. As you take the advice you've learned in this book and set out on the path toward a healthier heart, here are five tips to boost your chances of permanent success.

ASK THE EXPERT

Do some people just have more willpower than others? Is there anything you can do to increase your willpower?

Bess H. Marcus, Ph.D., professor of psychiatry and human behavior at the Brown University School of Medicine and coauthor of *Active Living Every Day*:

"It may be true that some people have more willpower than others. But my advice is not to get hung up on willpower. When you're trying to make lifelong changes, the point is not to depend on willpower—no matter whether you've got a little or a lot.

Here's why. When we say willpower, we typically mean something like being able to say no to the fudge brownies that someone passes around at work or having the strength to drive on by a fast-food restaurant even though you're hungry. And maybe you'll be able to do that now and then. But that's no way to live every day. The truth is, no matter how much willpower you've got, it's going to give out at some point—all the faster if that's all you depend on to make a healthy choice.

Instead, I like to think of willpower as something you keep in your back pocket, for the times you really need it. For everyday purposes, it's much better to depend on other, more reliable strategies.

Planning is one good example. Decide ahead of time where you're going to have lunch. Or pack a lunch that's healthy and low in calories. That way you don't have to use your willpower to drive past that fast-food restaurant. You can also avoid testing your willpower by putting temptation at arm's length. Don't even go near the dessert table, for instance.

Making sure you have options is another way to avoid depending on willpower. Let's say you normally walk for half an hour at lunch. If that's your only exercise option, and suddenly you have to decide whether to walk or to accept an invitation to go out with a friend, you have a crisis of willpower. But if you also have the option of walking after you get home from work or first thing in the morning, you aren't forced to make a hard decision that requires sheer willpower.

Of course there are certainly times when you will need to call on your willpower. And there are ways to make sure you've got enough when you need it. Getting enough sleep and controlling the stresses in your life are two important ones. It's hard to have willpower when you're feeling exhausted or totally stressed out. You'll also bolster your willpower by remembering why making the healthier choice is important to you.

But don't depend on it. And definitely don't use a lack of willpower as an excuse for not being able to adopt new health habits. The real reason people succeed at making lasting changes isn't because they have more willpower than someone else. It's really because they've learned skills and strategies that allow them to avoid relying on sheer willpower."

1. Have a game plan. Especially at the beginning, it's easy to feel overwhelmed by all the advice you hear and the changes you want to make. That's why it's important to have a plan for what you want to do—and how you intend to do it. The details should be a specific as you can make them. "Eating a healthier diet" just doesn't cut it. Instead, set a goal of eating at least six servings of fruits and vegetables a day. "Getting more exercise" doesn't make the grade, either. A better aim: putting in 40 minutes of walking or climbing on a stair machine five days a week.

Whatever goals you set, make sure they're realistic. We're not talking about a wish list; we're talking about an action plan. Decide on one or two concrete changes you want to make—then make them. Stick with them until you've successfully introduced the new habits, then tackle another.

Be sure to put your game plan in writing. Doing so represents a commitment—a contract with yourself. It should include both long-term goals and interim milestones along the way. One approach is to begin by thinking about where you want to be six months from now. Write down specific goals, such as "lose 20 pounds" or "exercise 5 times a week." Then break these goals into shorter-term targets for the next month. Finally, work out weekly plans for the coming month that will get you there. See "A Sample Heart Healthy Game Plan," opposite, for an idea of what an effective plan might look like.

2. Chart your progress. Once you have your plan drawn up, use a journal or notebook to keep track of your daily progress. The more closely you keep tabs, the better your chances of succeeding. Psychologists call this strategy self-monitoring, and it has proved a remarkably powerful motivational tool. Consider weight loss. Studies show that all people have to do is start keeping a food diary—a detailed accounting of what they eat every day—and they'll begin to lose weight, even if they don't consciously change anything else. Why? Keeping a food diary forces you to become more aware of everything you eat during the day. It also helps you spot simple changes you can make to help you meet your goal. Finally, charting your progress lets you know when you deserve a pat on the back.

TROUBLESHOOTING TIP

Adopting new habits is tough. One trick for making them stick is to practice them daily. Instead of walking for 40 minutes four or five times a week, for instance, aim to walk 30 minutes every single day—rain or shine. Making a daily commitment to yourself leaves less room for procrastination. And the more often you do something, the faster it becomes second nature.

A SAMPLE HEART HEALTHY GAME PLAN

In a notebook, write down your own heart health game plan using this one as a model. Start with the larger goals you want to accomplish. Next, list actions you're going to take this week. At the end of each week, note your progress. Then formulate your goals for the next week.

MY SIX-MONTH GOALS

1. Lose 20 pounds
2. Exercise 40 minutes a day
3. Eat at least six servings of fruits and vegetables a day

MY ONE-MONTH GOALS

1. Lose five pounds
2. Walk at least three times a week
3. Look into buying a stationary bike

MY GOALS FOR WEEK 1

1. Take three 15-minute walks this week
2. Have a glass of orange juice or a piece of fruit with cereal every morning
3. Switch from 2 percent to 1 percent milk

MY GOALS FOR WEEK 2

1. Take three 20-minute walks
2. Try at least one new low-calorie, low-fat recipe for dinner
3. Check out stationary bikes (rent vs. buy)

MY GOALS FOR WEEK 3

1. Take three 25-minute walks
2. Weigh myself to see how I'm doing
3. Fix two low-cal, low-fat recipes for dinner
4. Add a salad or vegetable side dish

MY GOALS FOR WEEK 4

1. Take three 30-minute walks
2. Fix low-fat recipes for dinner three times this week
3. Have a serving of fruit every morning for breakfast and at least two vegetables with dinner
4. Decide on a stationary bike

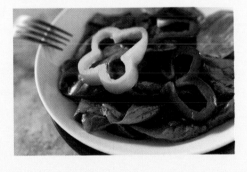

3. Find a friend. If doesn't matter whether you're trying to quit smoking, eat better, lose weight, exercise more, or all of the above. If you join forces with someone else who's trying to make the same changes, you'll dramatically improve your chances of success. A study at Indiana University revealed that people who exercise with a buddy are seven times more likely than those who go it alone to stick to their plan. And when researchers at St. George's Hospital Medical School in London paired up smokers trying to kick the habit, they found that the buddy system more than doubled their odds of quitting.

Who to enlist? Your spouse, another family member, a friend, or a coworker may be willing to join you. Many medical centers run support groups for people with heart disease—a great place to find others who want to make the same kind of lifestyle changes. Another option: Talk to your doctor. He or she may be able to put you in touch with other heart patients who are looking for company on the path to a healthier life. If you're looking for moral support, check out on-line resources, such as the American Heart Association's site at www.myheartwatch.com, which includes everything from personal stories from other patients to chat rooms and discussion groups.

4. Shake it up. One of the biggest stumbling blocks people face over the long term is boredom. If your exercise of choice is walking, you may find yourself getting tired of treading the same path day in and day out. Low-fat meals can be delicious; but if you turn to the same four or five recipes all the time, dinnertime is likely to get pretty monotonous.

If you start to feel bored, look for ways to make your new habits interesting again. Find a new place to walk. Better yet, take up a new activity. Challenge yourself by taking an exercise class or getting a new bicycle. Find a way to combine physical activity with something else you love. If you're an avid photographer, for example, take your camera along on walks and be on the lookout for great shots. If you're tired of the same old meals, get a new cookbook that features a cuisine you haven't tried before or sign up for a cooking class. Do you have friends who enjoy healthy cooking? Form a dinner club that allows you to try out new dishes together.

5. Keep your eyes on the prize. The only constant in life is change. As you move forward, keep in mind that the things that inspire you to action are likely to change. If you've had a heart attack, you may be motivated first by the fear of having another. As that

Key Finding

Men get more benefit from having an exercise buddy than women do, according to a 2001 study at Ohio State University. Women benefit more from family support. In a poll of 937 randomly selected students, men who exercised regularly reported that they had lots of support from friends who also exercised. Those who rarely worked out reported having few active friends. Physically active women, on the other hand, were much more likely to report being motivated by the encouragement of their families.

worry fades, you may find yourself encouraged by the desire to get your old energy back. Now and then, you may not feel very motivated at all. In fact, you may find yourself wondering if all the effort is really worth the trouble.

That's why it's so important to keep your eyes on the prize. Why have you decided to change for the better? To be healthier, of course. But what exactly does that mean? One measure of health is longevity. We'd all like to enjoy as many healthy years as we can. But since none of us knows how long our lives are meant to be, there's never a moment when we can say, hey, look, I'm enjoying the extra year or two I earned by living a healthier life.

Of course you'll probably be keeping an eye on other, more objective measures of health—things like weight and cholesterol and blood pressure. They're all important. But over time, they alone aren't usually powerful enough to keep people motivated.

What's the true reward of living a healthier life? In the end, it's how you feel every day. Having the energy to do the things you enjoy without getting tired or experiencing symptoms like shortness of breath or angina. Feeling stronger or more capable. Also a better mental outlook—being more in control, feeling more confident, enjoying the satisfaction that comes from accomplishing something you set your mind to do.

Some of the rewards you reap may surprise you. You may discover a satisfying hobby that involves a physical activity you never knew you enjoyed. You may learn to enjoy cooking more than you ever thought you could. By enlisting support from friends or coworkers, you may forge new or deeper relationships with others. By practicing relaxation techniques, you may develop a new sense of inner peace.

In the weeks and months to come, be conscious of all the rewards you experience, large and small. Take time to savor them. Your heart may be the reason you embarked on a healthier life. But you'll find plenty of other reasons to celebrate your new sense of well-being. And in turn, by appreciating all the benefits you enjoy, you'll find new sources of motivation and inspiration to keep you on the road to being heart healthy for life.

> "What's the true reward of living a healthier life? In the end, it's how you feel every day."

221

Recipes

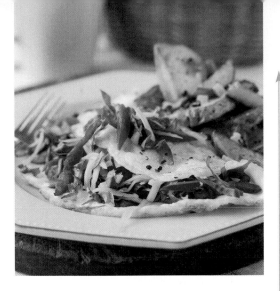

BREAKFAST

Egg-White Omelet With Vegetable- Cheddar Filling

More vegetables and less fat make this omelet a splendid way to start the day.

1 Serving

- 3 egg whites
- 1 teaspoon water
- 2 teaspoons chopped fresh dill (optional)
- 1/8 teaspoon salt
- 1/8 teaspoon freshly ground black pepper
- 1/2 cup loosely packed, thinly sliced fresh spinach
- 1 plum tomato, chopped
- 2 tablespoons shredded nonfat cheddar cheese

1. Whisk egg whites, 1 teaspoon water, dill (if using), salt, and pepper in medium bowl until soft peaks form. Toss spinach, tomato, and cheddar in small bowl.

2. Lightly coat nonstick omelet pan or small skillet with nonstick cooking spray and set over medium heat 1 minute. Pour egg mixture into pan and cook until eggs begin to set on bottom. Lift up edge of eggs with heat-proof spatula, pushing cooked part toward center of pan and letting uncooked portion run underneath. Cook until eggs are almost set and bottom is just lightly browned.

3. Spread filling over half of omelet, leaving 1/4-inch border and reserving 1 tablespoon mixture for garnish. Lift up omelet at edge nearest handle and fold in half, slightly off-center, so filling peeks out. Cook 2 minutes. Slide omelet onto plate and garnish with reserved filling.

NUTRITION INFORMATION
Per serving: 109 calories, 0.5 g total fat, 0 g saturated fat, 3 mg cholesterol, 1 g fiber, 18 g protein, 906 mg sodium

Whole-Grain Buttermilk Pancakes

Rich in whole grains that help lower your cholesterol, these have an appealing nutty flavor.

Makes 12 pancakes

- 2/3 cup unsifted whole-wheat flour
- 1/4 cup oat bran
- 1 tablespoon cornmeal
- 1 tablespoon brown sugar
- 1 1/2 teaspoons baking powder
- 1/4 teaspoon baking soda
- 1/4 teaspoon salt
- 1 cup buttermilk
- 2 large eggs, separated
- 2 tablespoons corn oil

1. In a medium-size bowl, combine whole-wheat flour, oat bran, cornmeal, sugar, baking powder, baking soda, and salt. In a 1-pint glass measuring cup, combine the buttermilk, egg yolks, and oil.

2. In a perfectly clean large bowl, beat the egg whites with an electric mixer set on high speed until they form stiff peaks. Stir the buttermilk mixture into the flour mixture. Fold in the egg whites.

3. Lightly coat a 12-inch nonstick skillet with the cooking spray and set over moderate heat. When the skillet is hot, cook the pancakes 4 at a time, using 1/4 cup batter for each. Cook for about 2 minutes on one side or until bubbles appear on the surface; turn, then cook 2 minutes longer or until golden brown on each side and cooked through.

NUTRITION INFORMATION
Per pancake: 76 calories, 4 g total fat, 1 g saturated fat, 36 mg cholesterol, 1 g fiber, 3 g protein, 36 mg sodium

Blueberry Sauce

Top your pancakes with either of these sauces, and you'll add a serving of fruit to your breakfast. They also make terrific toppings for frozen yogurt.

Makes 1⅓ cups

- ¾ **cup unsweetened apple juice**
- 4 **teaspoons honey**
- 1 **tablespoon cornstarch**
- ½ **teaspoon grated fresh ginger or ⅛ teaspoon ground ginger (optional)**
- 2 **cups blueberries or 1 package (12 ounces) frozen dry-pack blueberries, thawed**
- 1 **teaspoon lime or lemon juice**

1. In a small saucepan, stir together the apple juice, honey, cornstarch, and, if desired, ginger until the cornstarch dissolves. Add the blueberries, then bring to a simmer over moderate heat; cook, stirring, for 2 minutes. Remove from the heat and stir in the lime juice. Serve hot or warm.

NUTRITION INFORMATION
Per tablespoon: 18 calories, 0 g total fat, 0 g saturated fat, 0 mg cholesterol, 0 g fiber, 0 g protein, 1 mg sodium

Crushed Red Berry Sauce

Makes 1⅓ cups

- 1½ **cups thinly sliced strawberries or frozen dry-pack strawberries, thawed**
- 3 **tablespoons sugar**
- 1 **cup raspberries or frozen dry-pack raspberries, thawed**

1. In a medium-size bowl, sprinkle the strawberries with the sugar. Cover and let stand for 1 hour at room temperature, allowing the berries to form their own syrup.

2. Mash the strawberries with a potato masher or wooden spoon, then add the raspberries and mix well. Cover and refrigerate for at least 1 hour to let the flavors mellow. Serve chilled or at room temperature. Refrigerated, will keep for up to 5 days.

NUTRITION INFORMATION
Per tablespoon: 12 calories, 0 g total fat, 0 g saturated fat, 0 mg cholesterol, 1 g fiber, 0 g protein, 0 mg sodium

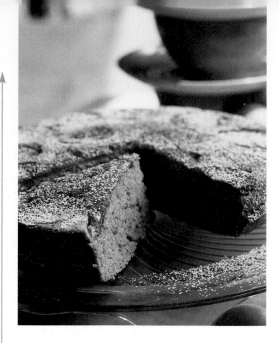

Apricot-Oat Breakfast Cake

This quick-to-make cake tastes too good to be true, but it boasts a host of heart healthy ingredients.

NOTE: You can buy oat flour in health food stores and some supermarkets. Or make it at home simply by processing rolled oats in a food processor until they are the texture of whole-wheat flour.

8 Servings

- ¾ **cup dried-apricot halves**
- 1 **cup boiling water**
- ½ **cup oat flour**
- ½ **cup all-purpose flour**
- ¼ **cup yellow cornmeal**
- ⅓ **cup firmly packed light brown sugar**
- 1 **teaspoon ground ginger**
- 1 **teaspoon baking powder**
- ½ **teaspoon baking soda**
- ½ **teaspoon salt**
- 1 **large egg plus 2 large egg whites**
- ½ **cup buttermilk**
- 2 **tablespoons extra light olive oil**
- 1½ **teaspoons confectioners' sugar**

1. Preheat oven to 350°F. Spray 8-inch round non-stick baking pan with nonstick cooking spray. Combine apricot halves and boiling water and let stand 15 minutes to soften. Drain apricots and arrange in bottom of pan.

2. Meanwhile, combine oat flour, all-purpose flour, cornmeal, brown sugar, ginger, baking powder, baking soda, and salt in medium bowl.

3. In separate bowl, stir together whole egg, egg whites, buttermilk, and olive oil. Make well in center of dry ingredients. Pour egg mixture into well, stirring just until moistened.

4. Pour batter over apricots and smooth top. Bake until cake tester inserted in center comes out clean, about 30 minutes. Cool on wire rack for 10 minutes. Turn cake out onto rack to cool completely. Dust with confectioners' sugar. Cut into 8 wedges.

NUTRITION INFORMATION
Per serving: 201 calories, 4.5 g total fat, 1 g saturated fat, 27 mg cholesterol, 2 g fiber, 5 g protein, 295 mg sodium

Salads

Fruity Tabbouleh

Loaded with fiber, this Mediterranean-inspired recipe helps lower cholesterol and stabilize blood sugar. It makes a delicious lunch.

4 Servings

- 1 **cup coarse bulgur (cracked wheat)**
- ½ **teaspoon salt**
- 2½ **cups boiling water**
- 1 **apple, cut into small dice**
- 1 **tablespoon fresh lemon juice**
- ½ **cup sliced almonds, lightly toasted**
- ½ **cup dried-apricot halves, cut into fine bits**
- 2 **green onions, very finely chopped (¼ cup)**
- 1 **tablespoon chopped fresh parsley**
- 1 **tablespoon chopped fresh mint**
- 1 **tablespoon canola oil or light olive oil**

1. Place the bulgur in a medium bowl. Stir in the salt. Cover with boiling water and set aside for 1 hour.

2. Meanwhile, in a large bowl, toss the apples in the lemon juice until well coated. Add the almonds, apricots, and onions. Mix the parsley and mint and stir in, along with the oil.

3. Drain the soaked bulgur if necessary. Toss and gently stir into the fruit mixture. Refrigerate for at least 1 hour or overnight. Serve chilled.

NUTRITION INFORMATION
Per serving: 283 calories, 10 g total fat, 1 g saturated fat, 0 mg cholesterol, 10 g fiber, 8 g protein, 302 mg sodium

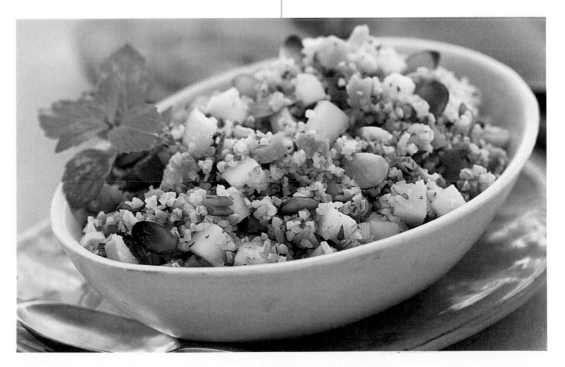

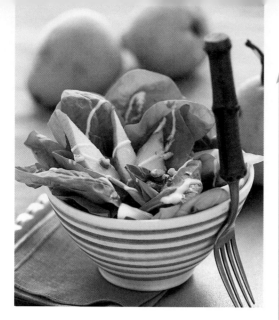

Spinach Salad with Pears and Walnuts

The yogurt dressing gives this simple salad a delightful tang.

4 Servings

- ¾ cup plain low-fat yogurt
- 1 clove garlic, crushed
- 1 tablespoon olive oil
- ¼ teaspoon Dijon mustard
- 1 pound spinach, rinsed, trimmed, and torn into bite-size pieces
- 1 ripe pear, cored and thinly sliced (1⅓ cups)
- ¼ cup coarsely chopped walnuts (1 ounce)

1. In a food processor or blender, whirl the yogurt, garlic, oil, and mustard for 30 to 60 seconds or until smooth. In a large bowl, combine the spinach, pear, and walnuts. Pour the dressing over the salad and toss until coated.

NUTRITION INFORMATION
Per serving: 153 calories, 9 g total fat, 1 g saturated fat, 1 mg cholesterol, 4 g fiber, 7 g protein, 131 mg sodium

Tex-Mex Black and White Bean Salad

If you're counting calories, count on this satisfying salad. Full of flavor, it's high in water and fiber but low in calories.

4 Servings (about 6 cups)

- 1 clove garlic, halved
- 1 can (15 ounces) black beans, drained and rinsed
- 1 can (15 ounces) white beans, drained and rinsed
- 1 can (8.25 ounces) no-salt-added whole kernel corn, drained and rinsed
- 1 small jalapeño pepper, cored, seeded, and finely chopped
- 2 ripe tomatoes (about 8 ounces each), cored, halved horizontally, seeded, and diced (about 2 cups)
- 1 cucumber, peeled, seeded, and diced
- 2 scallions, trimmed and finely chopped (about ¼ cup)
- 1½ teaspoons ground cumin
- 1 teaspoon salt
- ¼ teaspoon black pepper
- 3–4 tablespoons lime juice (3 to 4 limes)
- ¼ cup chopped fresh cilantro
- 4 packed cups shredded romaine lettuce, from 1 head

1. Rub a large bowl with the cut garlic. In the bowl, fold together the beans, corn, chile, tomatoes, cucumber, scallions, cumin, salt, and pepper. Fold in the lime juice, to taste.

2. Just before serving, fold in the cilantro. For each serving, spread 1 packed cup shredded romaine lettuce on a plate, and spoon about 1½ cups of the salad over the romaine.

NUTRITION INFORMATION
Per serving: 189 calories, 2 g total fat, 0 g saturated fat, 0 mg cholesterol, 10 g fiber, 10 g protein, 217 mg sodium

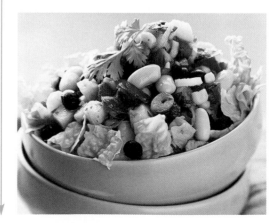

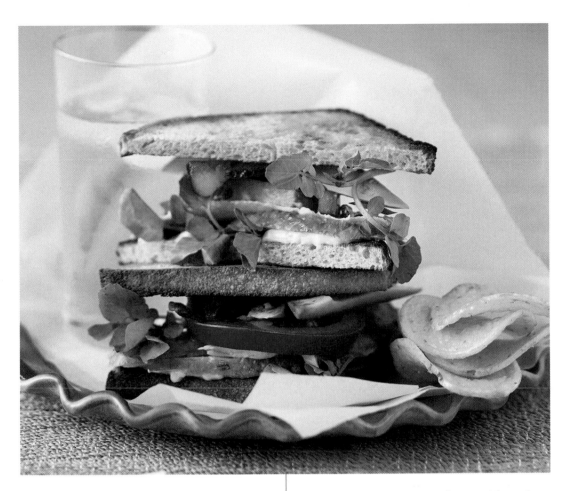

Sandwiches

Turkey Cobb Salad Sandwich

Hearty and healthful, this scrumptious sandwich squeezes in several vegetable servings. The avocado provides a dose of cholesterol-lowering monounsaturated fat.

4 Servings

- ¼ **cup nonfat mayonnaise**
- 1 **ounce blue cheese, crumbled (¼ cup)**
- 2 **tablespoons snipped fresh chives**
- 4 **slices lean bacon**
- 1 **small avocado**
- 8 **slices multigrain or sourdough bread, toasted**
- 4 **ounces watercress, tough stems trimmed**
- 12 **ounces fresh roasted turkey breast slices**
- 3 **medium tomatoes, sliced**
- 4 **scallions, thinly sliced**

1. Combine mayonnaise, blue cheese, and chives in small bowl.

2. Cook bacon in medium skillet over medium-high heat until crisp. Transfer to paper towels to drain, then tear into small pieces. Pit, peel, and thinly slice avocado.

3. Spread blue cheese mixture evenly on bread. Layer 4 slices with watercress, turkey, tomatoes, scallions, bacon, and avocado. Top with remaining bread and cut sandwiches diagonally in half.

NUTRITION INFORMATION
Per serving: 433 calories, 12 g total fat, 3 g saturated fat, 67 mg cholesterol, 5 g fiber, 36 g protein, 1,072 mg sodium

Tuna Provençale on A Baguette

You'll forget about eating fast food if you've packed this hearty sandwich in your brown bag. It's an easy way to get a helping of omega-3 fatty acids into your diet.

4 Servings

- **2 large tomatoes, peeled and chopped**
- **5 black olives, pitted and finely chopped**
- **¼ teaspoon salt**
- **1 baguette (6 ounces, about 24 inches long)**
- **1 ½ tablespoons extra-virgin olive oil**
- **1 large onion**
- **1 large green bell pepper**
- **2 cans (6 ounces each) water-packed albacore tuna, drained**
- **2 tablespoons white wine vinegar**
- **2 garlic cloves, minced**
- **¼ teaspoon anchovy paste**

1. Mix tomatoes, olives, and salt in medium bowl, and then let stand until juicy, about 15 minutes.

2. Meanwhile, cut bread almost in half lengthwise (do not slice completely through). Open like a book, being careful not to separate bread. Pull out about ½ cup of soft bready center with your hands. Using ½ tablespoon oil, brush cut sides of bread. Then spread on tomato mixture and any juices that have collected in bowl.

3. Cut onion in half through stem end, then cut crosswise into thin semicircles. Cut green pepper in half and then crosswise into thin semicircles. Layer onion, green pepper, and tuna over tomato mixture. Whisk vinegar, garlic, anchovy paste, and remaining oil in small bowl. Drizzle over tuna.

4. Wrap stuffed loaf tightly in plastic wrap. Weigh it down with heavy skillet and let stand at room temperature until ingredients have soaked into bread, about 30 minutes. Cut diagonally into 4 equal sandwiches.

NUTRITION INFORMATION
Per serving: 325 calories, 10 g total fat, 2 g saturated fat, 36 mg cholesterol, 4 g fiber, 26 g protein, 795 mg sodium

Soups

Tuscan Bean Soup

Colorful and incredibly rich in heart protective fiber, this soup is a meal in a bowl.

6 Servings

- **1 tablespoon olive oil**
- **2 medium onions, coarsely chopped**
- **2 medium carrots, coarsely chopped**
- **2 celery ribs, chopped**
- **2 cans (14½ ounces each) reduced-sodium chicken broth**
- **1 can (28 ounces) crushed tomatoes in puree**
- **½ cup chopped fresh basil**
- **2 tablespoons chopped fresh oregano or 1 teaspoon dried**
- **1 can (15½ ounces) red kidney beans**
- **1 can (15½ ounces) cannellini beans**
- **1 can (15½ ounces) chickpeas**
- **6 tablespoons freshly grated Parmesan cheese**

1. Heat oil in large nonstick Dutch oven over medium-high heat. Sauté onions, carrots, and celery until soft, about 5 minutes. Add broth, tomatoes in puree, basil, and oregano. Bring to a boil. Reduce heat to medium-low, partially cover, and cook 10 minutes.

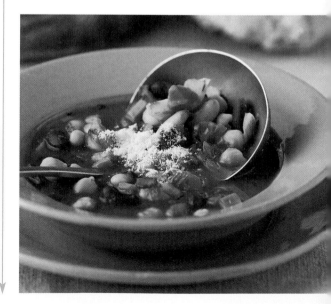

2. Put kidney and cannellini beans and chickpeas in colander; rinse and drain. Stir into soup. Cook until flavors develop, about 10 minutes more. Remove from heat.

3. Using an immersion blender, very coarsely puree about one-fourth of soup. Or transfer about 2 cups soup to food processor, very coarsely puree, and return to pot. Serve 2 cups soup per person topped with 1 tablespoon Parmesan.

NUTRITION INFORMATION
Per serving: 290 calories, 6 g total fat, 1.5 g saturated fat, 4 mg cholesterol, 10 g fiber, 15 g protein, 605 mg sodium

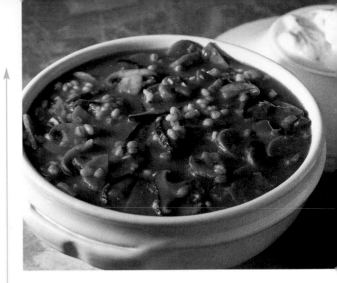

100-Calorie Chinese Chicken Soup

Broth-based soups fill you up on fewer calories. If you like tofu, you can substitute it for the chicken.

4 Servings

- **8** ounces boneless, skinned chicken breast halves, cut into bite-size pieces
- **2** teaspoons soy sauce
- **½** teaspoon Oriental sesame oil
- **2** cans (14½ ounces each) fat-free, reduced-sodium chicken broth
- **2** large cloves garlic, finely chopped
- **¼** teaspoon Chinese five-spice powder
- **1** small carrot, pared and thinly sliced
- **2** cups shredded spinach leaves (thick stems removed)
- **2** green onions, thinly sliced

1. In a small bowl, toss the chicken with the soy sauce and sesame oil. Set aside for 5 minutes.

2. In a large saucepan, heat the broth, garlic, and five-spice powder to a boil over medium heat.

3. Add the chicken with its juices and the carrot. Reduce the heat to medium-low and simmer for 5 minutes. Stir in the spinach and green onions. Simmer 1 minute longer. Serve hot.

NUTRITION INFORMATION
Per serving: 90 calories, 2 g total fat, 0 g saturated fat, 31 mg cholesterol, 1 g fiber, 13 g protein, 766 mg sodium

Old-Fashioned Mushroom Barley Soup

Barley is rich in cholesterol-lowering soluble fiber. Shiitake mushrooms add a depth of flavor to this otherwise old-fashioned soup.

4 Servings

- **2** teaspoons olive oil
- **1** onion, finely chopped
- **2** cloves garlic, minced
- **2** carrots, halved lengthwise and thinly sliced
- **¾** pound button mushrooms, sliced
- **¼** pound shiitake mushrooms, trimmed and thinly sliced
- **½** cup pearled barley
- **1** cup chicken broth
- **2** cups water
- **1** cup no-salt-added tomato sauce
- **¾** teaspoon each ground ginger and salt
- **½** teaspoon pepper

1. In a large saucepan, heat the oil over moderate heat. Add the onion and garlic and sauté for 5 minutes or until tender. Add the carrots and cook, stirring frequently, for 4 minutes or until crisp-tender. Add the button and shiitake mushrooms and cook, stirring frequently, for 5 minutes or until tender.

2. Stir in the barley, broth, 2 cups of water, the tomato sauce, ginger, salt, and pepper. Bring to a boil, reduce to a simmer, cover, and cook for 45 minutes or until the barley is tender.

NUTRITION INFORMATION
Per serving: 198 calories, 4 g total fat, 1 g saturated fat, 0 mg cholesterol, 8 g fiber, 7 g protein, 707 mg sodium

Chunky Gazpacho with Garlicky Croutons

A perfect summer supper, this chilled soup is bursting with vegetables and lean on calories and fat.

4 Servings

- 2 garlic cloves, peeled
- 4 slices French bread (1 inch thick)
- 1 teaspoon pepper
- ½ teaspoon salt
- ½ cup coarsely chopped red onion
- 1 can (28 ounces) no-salt-added tomatoes
- ¼ cup seasoned dry bread crumbs
- ¼ cup chopped parsley
- 3 tablespoons red wine vinegar
- 1 tablespoon olive oil
- 2 medium cucumbers, peeled and chopped
- 2 medium green bell peppers, chopped
- 2 medium red bell peppers, chopped

1. Preheat oven to 350°F. Cut 1 garlic clove in half and rub cut sides on inside of large bowl and on both sides of bread slices. Tear bread into 1-inch pieces. Put in the large bowl and lightly coat with nonstick cooking spray. Sprinkle with ½ teaspoon pepper and ¼ teaspoon salt. Toss to coat and transfer to a baking sheet. Bake croutons until golden, about 15 minutes. Cool completely.

2. Pulse onion and remaining garlic in food processor or blender until finely chopped. Add half of tomatoes and all their juice. Puree. Add bread crumbs, parsley, vinegar, oil, and remaining pepper and salt. Process just until blended and pour into large nonreactive bowl.

3. Chop remaining tomatoes. Stir into tomato mixture with half of chopped cucumbers and half of green and red peppers. Refrigerate until chilled, 1 hour. Ladle into bowls and top with remaining cucumber, green and red peppers, and croutons.

NUTRITION INFORMATION
Per serving: 250 calories, 5 g total fat, 1 g saturated fat, 0 mg cholesterol, 6 g fiber, 8 g protein, 730 mg sodium

Dinner

Pork Tenderloin With Honey-Mustard Sauce

Pork tenderloin is one of the leanest cuts of meat. This tender, tasty dish is ideal for entertaining.

4 Servings

- 1 tablespoon chopped fresh rosemary or 1 teaspoon dried
- 2 garlic cloves, minced
- 1 teaspoon grated lemon zest
- ½ teaspoon salt
- 1 pork tenderloin (about 1 pound), trimmed
- ⅓ cup fresh lemon juice
- ¼ cup honey
- 3 tablespoons coarse Dijon mustard
- ½ cup nonfat half-and-half
- 1 tablespoon all-purpose flour

1. Preheat oven to 400°F. Line small roasting pan with foil. Combine rosemary, garlic, lemon zest, and salt in small bowl and rub evenly over pork tenderloin; transfer pork to pan. Mix lemon juice, honey, and mustard in small bowl. Transfer half to small saucepan and set aside.

2. Brush pork with 2 tablespoons honey-mustard sauce. Roast pork until glazed and golden brown or until instant-read thermometer registers 160°F, about 25 minutes, basting 2 or 3 times with remaining sauce.

3. Meanwhile, put half-and-half in small bowl and whisk in flour until smooth. Warm reserved honey-mustard sauce in small saucepan over low heat. Gradually whisk in half-and-half mixture and cook, whisking constantly, until sauce thickens, about 3 minutes. Serve with pork.

NUTRITION INFORMATION
Per serving: 247 calories, 5 g total fat, 1 g saturated fat, 74 mg cholesterol, 1 g fiber, 25 g protein, 525 mg sodium

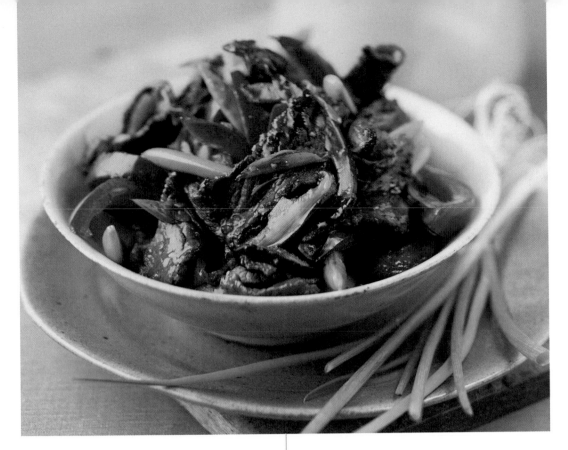

Garden Beef Stir-Fry With Hoisin Sauce

Much more healthful than Chinese takeout, this recipe skimps on oil but not on flavor.

4 Servings

- 12 ounces lean beef sirloin steak
- 2 tablespoons low-sodium teriyaki sauce
- 10 medium shiitake mushrooms
- 8 ounces sugar snap peas or snow peas
- 2 large red bell peppers
- 1 ½ cups low-sodium chicken broth or water
- 3 tablespoons hoisin sauce
- 2 tablespoons cornstarch
- 1 tablespoon vegetable oil
- 4 scallions, thinly sliced, diagonally
- 2 garlic cloves, crushed

1. If desired, put steak in freezer for 20 minutes to chill for easier slicing. Cut beef across grain into strips, about ⅛ inch thick, then halve extra-long pieces crosswise. Toss beef with teriyaki sauce in medium bowl. Cover and refrigerate at least 15 minutes or up to several hours.

2. Meanwhile, prepare vegetables: Discard stems from mushrooms. Thinly slice caps. Trim ends from peas and remove strings with fingers. Cut red peppers into thin strips. Blend ¼ cup broth, hoisin sauce, and cornstarch until smooth. Set aside.

3. Heat 1 teaspoon oil in large nonstick skillet or wok over high heat until hot but not smoking. Add scallions and stir-fry 1 minute. Transfer to large bowl. Add beef and garlic to skillet and stir-fry until beef is no longer pink, about 2 minutes. Transfer to bowl with scallions. Add another teaspoon oil to skillet. Stir-fry mushrooms until they begin to soften, about 3 minutes, and then transfer to bowl with beef mixture. Add remaining oil and stir-fry snap peas and red peppers just until they begin to soften, 1 to 2 minutes.

4. Return beef and vegetables to skillet and stir in remaining broth. Cover and cook over medium heat until all ingredients are heated through but vegetables are still crisp-tender, 2 to 3 minutes. Whisk hoisin sauce mixture and pour into skillet. Stir-fry until sauce boils, and then cook 1 minute longer.

NUTRITION INFORMATION
Per serving: 263 calories, 8.5 g total fat, 2 g saturated fat, 48 mg cholesterol, 5 g fiber, 21 g protein, 543 mg sodium

Turkey Burgers with Fresh Pineapple Salsa

A secret heart healthy ingredient keeps these burgers moist and flavorful. The Caribbean-inspired salsa is a sweet way to add another fruit serving to your day's tally.

4 Servings

- 1 **small pineapple**
- 1 **small mango, peeled and finely chopped**
- 1 **small red onion, minced**
- 2 **tablespoons finely chopped fresh cilantro**
- 1 **tablespoon fresh lemon juice**
- 1 **teaspoon vegetable oil**
- 12 **ounces ground skinless turkey breast**
- 1 **large Granny Smith apple, peeled and shredded**
- ¼ **cup seasoned dry bread crumbs**
- 4 **thin slices reduced-fat American cheese (½ ounce each)**
- 4 **hamburger buns or soft rolls, split**
    Green leaf lettuce

1. Peel, core, slice, and chop pineapple (you need 2 cups); put into medium bowl. Mix in mango, onion, cilantro, lemon juice, and oil. Cover and set aside.

2. Mix turkey, apple, and bread crumbs in another medium bowl until blended. Divide mixture into 4 equal portions and shape into burgers about ½ inch thick. Place burgers on a plate, cover, and put into freezer until chilled, about 20 minutes.

3. Meanwhile, preheat grill to medium or preheat broiler. Cook burgers 8 inches from heat until browned and cooked through, about 8 minutes on each side.

4. For each sandwich, place a slice of cheese on bottom of bun, cover with lettuce, add burger, top with about ½ cup salsa, and crown with top of bun.

NUTRITION INFORMATION
Per serving: 383 calories, 5 g total fat, 1.5 g saturated fat, 66 mg cholesterol, 4 g fiber, 32 g protein, 701 mg sodium

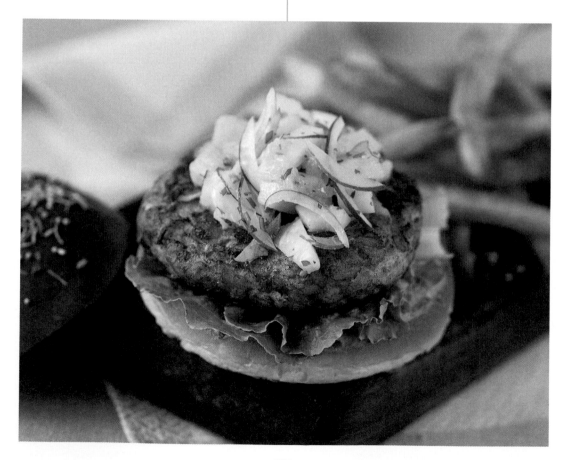

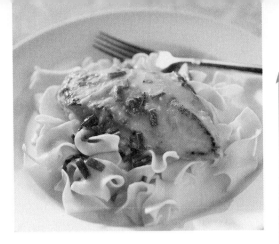

Chicken Breasts in Garlic Butter with Chives

Roasting gives the heart healthy garlic a mellow flavor in this richly satisfying recipe. Serve over pasta to soak up the sauce.

4 Servings

- 1 **head of garlic (2 ounces)**
- ²⁄₃ **cup chicken broth**
- 1 **teaspoon grated lemon zest**
- 1 **tablespoon fresh lemon juice**
- ¼ **teaspoon salt**
- ¼ **teaspoon freshly ground black pepper**
- 2 **teaspoons olive oil**
- 4 **skinless, boneless chicken breast halves (about 1½ pounds)**
- 2 **tablespoons flour**
- 1 **tablespoon butter, cut up**
- ¼ **cup snipped chives**

1. Preheat oven to 400°F. Wrap garlic in foil and bake for 30 minutes or until packet feels soft when squeezed. When cool enough to handle, remove foil, snip off top of head of garlic, and squeeze garlic pulp into small bowl. Whisk broth, lemon zest, lemon juice, salt, and pepper into garlic; set aside.

2. Meanwhile, in large nonstick skillet, heat oil over medium heat. Dredge chicken in flour, shaking off excess. Add chicken to pan and sauté 4 minutes per side or until golden brown. With slotted spoon, transfer chicken to plate.

3. Whisk garlic mixture to combine and pour into skillet. Bring to a boil, return chicken to pan, reduce to a simmer, cover, and cook 5 minutes or until chicken is cooked through. Transfer chicken to dinner plates.

4. Return sauce to a simmer. Remove from heat and swirl in butter until creamy. Stir in chives and spoon sauce over chicken.

NUTRITION INFORMATION
Per serving: 272 calories, 7.5 g total fat, 2.5 g saturated fat, 107 mg cholesterol, 41 g protein, 461 mg sodium

Barbecued Fish Steaks

The tangy sauce is sure to make this fish a hit. And it's such a snap to prepare, you can easily serve it during the week.

4 Servings

- 3 **small scallions**
- ¼ **cup reduced-sodium soy sauce**
- ⅓ **cup apricot jam**
- 3 **tablespoons ketchup**
- 1 **tablespoon red wine vinegar**
- 4 **halibut steaks (6 ounces each)**

1. Preheat broiler. Thinly slice scallions on diagonal. Set aside.

2. Combine soy sauce, jam, ketchup, and vinegar in small bowl. Measure out ⅓ cup of mixture and set aside as a sauce.

3. Place halibut steaks on broiler rack and brush with remaining soy mixture. Broil 4 inches from heat until browned and cooked through, about 5 minutes.

4. Spoon reserved sauce over fish. Pass a small bowl of sliced scallions at table for sprinkling over fish.

NUTRITION INFORMATION
Per serving: 164 calories, 4 g total fat, 1 g saturated fat, 0 mg cholesterol, 5 g fiber, 11 g protein, 681 mg sodium

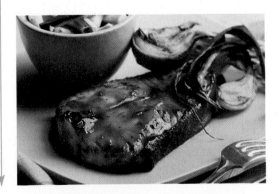

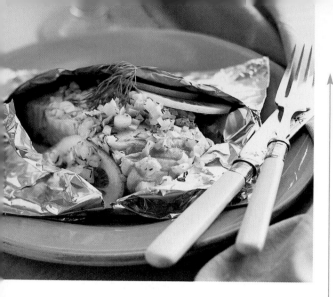

Foil-Baked Salmon with Lemon and Dill

Here's a simple, delicious way to serve salmon, which is bursting with omega-3 fatty acids and may help lower your risk of a heart attack.

4 Servings

- 4 **salmon fillets (6 ounces each)**
- ½ **teaspoon salt**
- ⅛ **teaspoon pepper**
- ¼ **cup finely chopped green onion**
- ¼ **cup finely chopped fresh dill or**
- 2 **tablespoons dried dill**
- 8 **thin slices lemon**
- ¼ **cup water, fish bouillon, or chicken broth**

1. Place a baking sheet on the middle rack in the oven and preheat the oven to 400°F.

2. Tear off 8 sheets of aluminum foil, each 12 x 12 inches. Using a double layer of foil, place each salmon fillet in the center of a foil square. Sprinkle evenly with salt and pepper. Combine the green onion and dill in a small cup. Sprinkle evenly over the fillets. Top with lemon slices. Drizzle each fillet with 1 tablespoon of the water, bouillon, or broth.

3. Seal each packet by bringing two opposite sides of the foil up and over the fish. Fold the edges over twice, then fold the side edges twice. Place the packets on the preheated baking sheet.

NUTRITION INFORMATION
Per serving: 192 calories, 6 g total fat, 1 g saturated fat, 83 mg cholesterol, 1 g fiber, 32 g protein, 399 mg sodium

Fried Rice with Tofu And Vegetables

Tofu helps bring cholesterol under control, and in this dish it absorbs the flavor of the sweet and savory sauce.

4 Servings

- 1 **cup dry white wine or chicken broth**
- ¼ **cup light soy sauce**
- 2 **tablespoons honey**
- 1 **tablespoon grated peeled fresh ginger**
- 12 **ounces extra-firm tofu, cut into ½-inch cubes**
- 1 **cup long-grain white rice**
- 2 **garlic cloves, minced**
- 1 **package (16 ounces) frozen mixed Chinese vegetables, slightly thawed**
- 5 **scallions, cut into 2-inch pieces**
- ¼ **teaspoon pepper**
- 1 **large egg, lightly beaten**

1. Put wine or broth, 1 tablespoon soy sauce, honey, and 1 teaspoon ginger in zip-close plastic bag. Add tofu, push out excess air, close, and shake gently to coat. Marinate in refrigerator 1 hour, turning occasionally.

2. Cook rice according to package directions; keep warm. Meanwhile, lightly coat wok or large deep skillet with nonstick cooking spray and set over high heat until hot but not smoking.

3. Stir-fry garlic and remaining ginger until fragrant, about 1 minute. Add mixed vegetables, half of scallions, rice, remaining soy sauce, and pepper. Stir-fry until mixed vegetables are heated through, about 4 minutes. Push ingredients to one side of wok, and then pour in beaten egg. Cook egg until almost set, cutting egg into strips with heat-proof spatula.

4. Pour marinade into small saucepan. Boil over high heat 2 minutes. Add tofu and marinade to wok. Stir-fry until tofu is heated through, about 4 minutes. Sprinkle with remaining scallions.

NUTRITION INFORMATION
Per serving: 442 calories, 9 g total fat, 2 g saturated fat, 53 mg cholesterol, 3 g fiber, 21 g protein, 668 mg sodium

Baked Macaroni with Four Cheeses

Everyone loves macaroni and cheese, and this lower-fat version lets you enjoy it without concern. The cheese supplies calcium, which helps control high blood pressure.

8 Servings

- 1 **pound elbow macaroni**
- 2 **large onions, chopped**
- 4 **cups nonfat half-and-half**
- ¼ **cup all-purpose flour**
- 2 **teaspoons dry mustard**
- ¼ **teaspoon salt**
- ½ **teaspoon pepper**
- 2 **cups shredded reduced-fat cheddar cheese (8 ounces)**
- 1½ **cups shredded part-skim mozzarella cheese (6 ounces)**
- ½ **cup shredded reduced-fat Monterey Jack cheese (2 ounces)**
- 8 **ounces nonfat cream cheese**
- 1½ **teaspoons paprika**

1. Preheat oven to 350°F. Lightly coat 13- x 9-inch baking dish with nonstick cooking spray. Cook macaroni according to package directions; drain and set aside.

2. Meanwhile, coat large saucepan with cooking spray and set over medium-high heat. Sauté onions until soft, about 5 minutes. Put ½ cup half-and-half and flour into jar with tight-fitting lid and shake until blended and smooth. Stir into onions in skillet, then blend in remaining half-and-half. Whisk in mustard, salt, and pepper and bring to a simmer. Continue cooking, whisking constantly, until mixture thickens, about 3 minutes.

3. Add cheddar, mozzarella, Monterey Jack, and cream cheese. Cook, stirring, until cheeses melt. Remove from heat and fold in macaroni. Spoon mixture into baking dish and sprinkle with paprika. Bake until bubbly and lightly browned, about 35 minutes.

NUTRITION INFORMATION
Per serving: 484 calories, 8 g total fat, 5 g saturated fat, 25 mg cholesterol, 2 g fiber, 29 g protein, 669 mg sodium

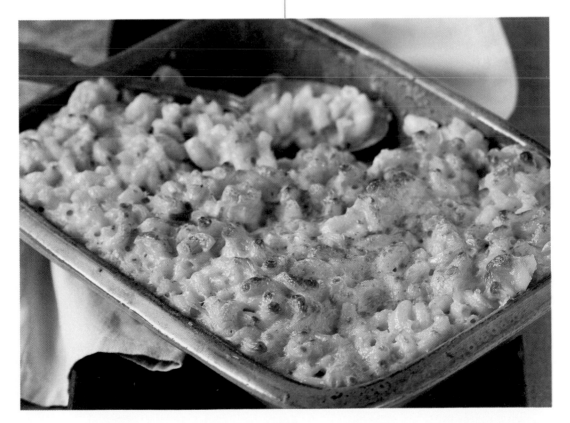

Vegetable Couscous

Find out just how satisfying a meatless meal can be with this hearty recipe.

4 to 6 Servings

- **2 tablespoons olive oil**
- **2 medium-size yellow onions, thinly sliced (4 cups)**
- **2 large carrots, peeled and sliced ½ inch thick**
- **2 medium-size red-skinned potatoes (6 ounces each), cut into ½-inch cubes**
- **3 cloves garlic, minced**
- **4 cups chicken stock, vegetable stock, or low-sodium chicken broth**
- **1 can (14½ ounces) low-sodium tomatoes, chopped, with their juice**
- **½ teaspoon each dried thyme and basil, crumbled**
- **½ teaspoon each salt and black pepper, or to taste**
- **1 bay leaf**
- **2 parsnips (7 ounces), peeled and sliced ½ inch thick**
- **1 medium-size zucchini (6 ounces), cut into 1-inch cubes**
- **1 medium-size yellow squash (6 ounces), cut into 1-inch cubes**
- **2 cups cooked chickpeas**
- **¼ cup golden raisins**
- **1 cup couscous**

1. In a 5-quart Dutch oven, heat 1 tablespoon of the oil over moderate heat. Add the onions and sauté, stirring occasionally, for 5 to 7 minutes or until golden. Add the carrots, potatoes, and garlic and cook, stirring, for 2 minutes. Stir in the stock or broth, tomatoes, thyme, basil, salt, pepper, and bay leaf. Bring the liquid to a boil, then lower the heat and simmer the vegetables, covered, for 5 minutes. Add the parsnips and simmer, covered, for 3 minutes. Add the zucchini, yellow squash, and chickpeas and simmer, covered, for 8 minutes or until the vegetables are just tender. Remove and discard the bay leaf.

2. Using a 1-pint glass measuring cup, transfer 1½ cups of the cooking liquid from the Dutch oven to a small saucepan. Stir in the raisins and the remaining 1 tablespoon of oil, then bring the liquid

to a boil and stir in the couscous. Remove the saucepan from the heat and let stand, covered, for 10 minutes or until the liquid is absorbed and the couscous is tender. Serve the vegetables over the couscous.

NUTRITION INFORMATION
Per serving: 570 calories, 11 g total fat, 1 g saturated fat, 0 mg cholesterol, 14 g fiber, 20 g protein, 453 mg sodium

Orecchiette with Cannellini Beans and Arugula

Beans, vegetables, and pasta come together deliciously in this nutrition-packed meal.

4 Servings

- **12 ounces orecchiette pasta**
- **8 ounces arugula**
- **1 small carrot, grated**
- **1 small red onion, chopped**
- **3 garlic cloves, minced**
- **1 can (28 ounces) plum tomatoes in puree**
- **1 cup reduced-sodium chicken broth**

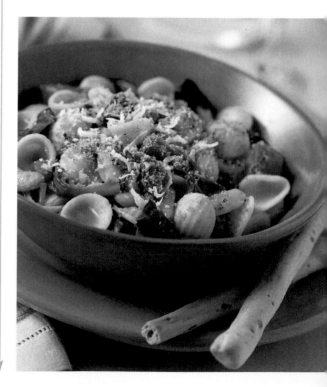

- 1 **can (15½ ounces) cannellini beans, rinsed and drained**
- ¼ **cup chopped basil**
- ¼ **cup grated Parmesan cheese**
- ½ **teaspoon salt**
- ¼ **cup seasoned dry bread crumbs**

1. Cook pasta according to package directions. Drain and keep warm.

2. Meanwhile, wash arugula well, remove any tough stems, and tear into bite-size pieces. Lightly coat Dutch oven with nonstick cooking spray and place over medium-high heat. Sauté carrot, onion, and garlic until tender, about 5 minutes.

3. Add tomatoes in puree, broth, beans, 2 table-spoons basil, 2 tablespoons Parmesan, and salt. Simmer, uncovered, 5 minutes. Add arugula and cook until sauce is bubbling, about 4 minutes. Mix in pasta and heat through, about 2 minutes. Transfer to pasta bowl. Sprinkle with bread crumbs and remaining basil and Parmesan.

NUTRITION INFORMATION
Per serving: 489 calories, 4 g total fat, 1 g saturated fat, 4 mg cholesterol, 9 g fiber, 21 g protein, 826 mg sodium

Vegetables

Roasted Harvest Vegetables

Full of fiber, roasted vegetables make a terrific complement to any fall or winter meal.

4 Servings

- 3 **tablespoons olive oil**
- 6 **cloves garlic, sliced**
- 3 **cups chunks (1-inch) butternut squash**
- 10 **ounces brussels sprouts, trimmed and halved lengthwise**
- 8 **ounces fresh shiitake mushrooms, stems discarded and caps thickly sliced**
- 2 **large red apples (unpeeled), cut into 1-inch chunks**
- ¼ **cup oil-packed sun-dried tomatoes, drained and thinly sliced**

- 1 **teaspoon dried rosemary, minced**
- ½ **teaspoon salt**
- ¼ **cup grated Parmesan cheese**

1. Preheat the oven to 400°F. In a large roasting pan, combine the olive oil and garlic. Heat for 3 minutes in the oven. Add the squash, brussels sprouts, mushrooms, apples, sun-dried tomatoes, rosemary, and salt; toss to combine.

2. Roast for 35 minutes, or until the vegetables are tender; toss the vegetables every 10 minutes. Sprinkle the Parmesan over the vegetables and roast for 5 minutes longer.

NUTRITION INFORMATION
Per serving: 292 calories, 14 g total fat, 2 g saturated fat, 4 mg cholesterol, 9.3 g fiber, 8 g protein, 464 mg sodium

Carrots with Orange-Ginger Glaze

A simple glaze turns the everyday carrot into an elegant side dish.

4 Servings

- 1 **teaspoon grated orange rind**
- ¾ **cup orange juice**
- 1½ **teaspoons unsalted butter or margarine**
- 1 **teaspoon honey**
- ½ **teaspoon ground ginger**
- ¼ **teaspoon salt**
- ⅛ **teaspoon black pepper**
- 4 **large carrots, peeled and cut diagonally into ½-inch slices (about 5 cups)**

1. In a 10-inch nonstick skillet, combine the orange rind, orange juice, butter, honey, ginger, salt, and pepper and bring to a boil. Add the carrots, lower the heat, and simmer, covered, for 5 minutes or until the carrots are slightly tender but still firm.

2. Raise the heat to high and boil the mixture, uncovered, shaking the pan frequently, for 5 min-utes or until the liquid has reduced to 3 table-spoons and the carrots are crisp-tender and nicely glazed.

NUTRITION INFORMATION
Per serving: 74 calories, 2 g total fat, 1 g saturated fat, 4 mg cholesterol, 3 g fiber, 1 g protein, 165 mg sodium

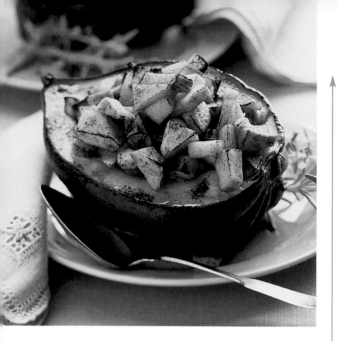

Cider-Baked Acorn Squash with Apple Stuffing

High in water content, squash provides bulk without a lot of calories. Enjoy this as a side dish, and you'll check off at least one serving of vegetables and one serving of fruit.

4 Servings

- 2 small acorn squash (about 1 pound each), halved lengthwise and seeded
- ½ cup apple cider or apple juice
- ½ teaspoon salt
- 1 apple pared, cored, and chopped
- 1 tablespoon light-brown sugar
- ¼ teaspoon cinnamon
- ⅛ teaspoon nutmeg

1. Preheat the oven to 350°F.

2. Place the squash halves cut-side down in a 13- x 9-inch baking dish. Add the cider to the pan.

3. Bake in the preheated oven for 30 minutes. Remove the pan from the oven and leave the oven on. Carefully turn the squash cut-side up and sprinkle with salt.

4. Combine the apple, sugar, cinnamon, and nutmeg in a small bowl. Spoon this mixture evenly into the squash halves. Drizzle the cider from the baking pan over the mixture, using a baster if you have one. Add a couple of spoonfuls of water to the pan.

5. Bake the squash, stuffed-side up, for 30 minutes longer or until tender.

NUTRITION INFORMATION
Per serving: 123 calories, 0 g total fat, 0 g saturated fat, 0 mg cholesterol, 7 g fiber, 2 g protein, 298 mg sodium

Grilled Summer Vegetables

Team these flavorful veggies with grilled fish for a palate-pleasing meal.

4 Servings

- 2 small fennel bulbs (about 8 ounces each), cleaned
- 1 small eggplant (about 1 pound), cut lengthwise into 2 slices ½ inch thick
- 4 plum tomatoes, halved
- 3 large bell peppers (preferably 1 green, 1 red, 1 yellow), cut into strips ½ inch wide
- ½ teaspoon salt
- ½ teaspoon pepper
- 2 tablespoons orange juice
- 8 basil leaves, slivered
- 1 garlic clove, minced
- 1 teaspoon grated orange zest

1. Preheat grill to high. Prepare fennel: Cut off stalks with fronds and set aside. Peel bulbs and cut vertically into ½-inch slices. Coat fennel, eggplant, tomatoes, and bell peppers with nonstick cooking spray (preferably olive-oil flavored) and sprinkle with salt and pepper.

2. Grill vegetables until tender and evenly browned, about 4 minutes on each side, turning once. Transfer to serving platter and sprinkle with orange juice.

3. Finely chop 1 tablespoon reserved fennel fronds and mix in small bowl with basil, garlic, and orange zest. Sprinkle over vegetables. Serve vegetables warm or at room temperature.

NUTRITION INFORMATION
Per serving: 118 calories, 1 g total fat, 0 g saturated fat, 0 mg cholesterol, 9 g fiber, 4 g protein, 364 mg sodium

Snacks

Guacamole with a Kick

This is lighter than traditional guacamole but packs plenty of flavor—along with cholesterol-lowering monounsaturated fat.

Makes 3 cups

- ½ **cup low-fat plain yogurt**
- 2 **small jalapeño peppers**
- 2 **plum tomatoes, finely chopped**
- 1 **small white onion, finely chopped**
- 2 **tablespoons minced cilantro**
- ½ **teaspoon salt**
- ½ **cup nonfat sour cream**
- 2 **large avocados**
- 2 **tablespoons fresh lime juice**
- 3 **ounces baked tortilla chips**

1. Line bottom of strainer with cheesecloth, coffee filter, or paper towel and set over medium bowl (strainer should not touch bottom of bowl). Spoon in yogurt, cover, and refrigerate 8 hours or overnight, until yogurt cheese is thick and creamy.

2. Remove seeds and ribs from jalapeños with

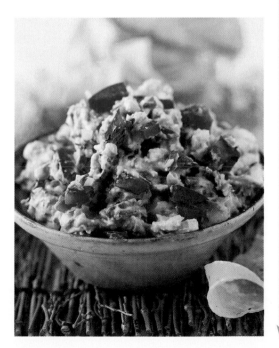

melon baller (wear gloves when handling, as the peppers can burn); mince. Mix jalapeños, tomatoes, onion, cilantro, and salt in large bowl. Fold in yogurt cheese and sour cream.

3. Halve, pit, and peel the avocados. Mash with a potato masher and sprinkle with the lime juice. Quickly fold into the tomato mixture. Serve with baked tortilla chips.

NUTRITION INFORMATION
Per serving (3 tablespoons): 72 calories, 4 g total fat, 0.75 g saturated fat, 0 mg cholesterol, 2 g fiber, 2 g protein, 124 mg sodium

Pumpkin-Date Muffins With Almonds

These tender, slightly sweet muffins have it all: dates for fiber, almonds for heart healthy unsaturated fats, and pumpkin for antioxidant power.

Makes 12 muffins

- 1½ **cups flour**
- ⅓ **cup packed light brown sugar**
- 2 **teaspoons baking powder**
- ½ **teaspoon baking soda**
- ¼ **teaspoon salt**
- ½ **cup chopped dates**
- ¼ **cup chopped almonds**
- 1 **cup canned solid-pack pumpkin purée**
- 2 **eggs, lightly beaten**
- ½ **cup low-fat (1.5 percent) buttermilk**
- ½ **cup reduced-fat sour cream**

1. Preheat the oven to 350°F. Line a 2½-inch muffin tin with paper liners. In a large bowl, stir together the flour, brown sugar, baking powder, baking soda, and salt. Stir in the dates and almonds.

2. In a medium bowl, combine the pumpkin, eggs, buttermilk, and sour cream. Make a well in the center of the dry ingredients and pour in the pumpkin mixture. Stir just until combined. Spoon into the prepared muffin cups and bake for 30 to 35 minutes or until a cake tester inserted in the center comes out clean.

NUTRITION INFORMATION
Per muffin: 157 calories, 4 g total fat, 1 g saturated fat, 39 mg cholesterol, 2 g fiber, 5 g protein, 204 mg sodium

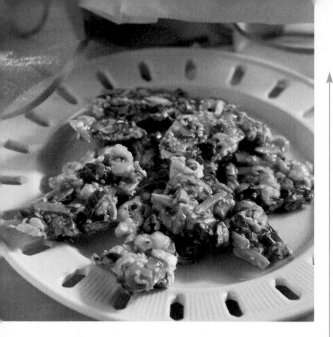

Almond Brittle

Instead of a candy bar, try this delicious snack loaded with heart healthy almonds.

Makes 1 pound 2 ounces

- 1 **cup whole natural almonds, coarsely chopped**
- 1/3 **cup slivered almonds**
- 3 **tablespoons sesame seeds**
- 1 **cup sugar**
- 1/2 **cup light corn syrup**
- 1/3 **cup water**
- 1 **teaspoon vanilla extract**
- 1/4 **teaspoon baking soda**
- 1 **tablespoon unsalted butter**
- 1 **cup air-popped popcorn**

1. Preheat the oven to 350°F. Toast the chopped and slivered almonds for 5 minutes or until golden brown. In a separate pan, toast the sesame seeds for 5 minutes or until lightly browned. Spray a large baking sheet with nonstick cooking spray; set aside.

2. In a medium saucepan, combine the sugar, corn syrup, and 1/3 cup of water. Cook over moderately high heat, stirring until the sugar has dissolved. Continue to cook, without stirring, for 7 minutes or until the sugar mixture reaches 290°F on a candy thermometer.

3. Immediately remove from the heat and stir in the vanilla, baking soda, and butter. Working as

quickly as possible, add the almonds, sesame seeds, and popcorn, stirring to coat. Quickly transfer to the prepared pan and use an oiled metal spatula to spread the brittle as flat as possible before it begins to harden. Cool to room temperature, then break the brittle into bite-size pieces.

NUTRITION INFORMATION
Per ounce: 132 calories, 7 g total fat, 1 g saturated fat, 2 mg cholesterol, 1 g fiber, 2 g protein, 30 mg sodium

Spiced Walnuts

Serve these as a spicy snack in place of chips at your next gathering.

12 1-ounce servings

- 1 **tablespoon oil**
- 2 **cups walnut halves**
- 3 **tablespoons sugar**
- 1/2 **teaspoon salt**
- 1/2 **teaspoon cayenne pepper**

1. In large heavy skillet, heat oil over moderate heat. Add walnut halves, tossing to coat. Add sugar, salt, and cayenne pepper and cook, stirring constantly, for 8 minutes or until nuts are well coated and sugar has caramelized. Serve hot or at room temperature.

NUTRITION INFORMATION
Per serving: 129 calories, 12 g fat, 98 mg sodium

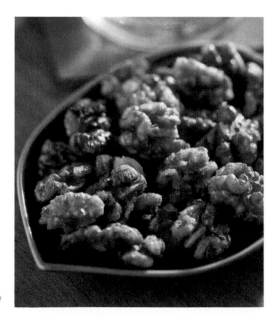

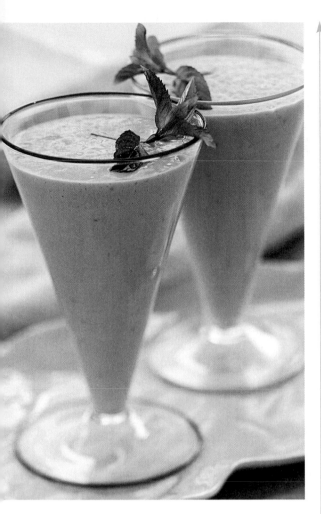

Tropical Soy Smoothie

This creamy drink's a fun, refreshing way to add some soy to your diet.

1 Serving

- ¼ **cup pineapple cubes**
- ¼ **cup mango cubes**
- 2 **strawberries, hulled**
- 1 **cup plain low-fat soy milk**
  Juice of ½ lime (1 tablespoon)

1. Combine the pineapple, mango, strawberries, soy milk, and lime juice in the container of a blender or food processor. Whirl until smooth, stopping to scrape down the sides of the container if necessary. Pour into a tall glass.

NUTRITION INFORMATION
Per serving: 193 calories, 3 g total fat, 0 g saturated fat, 0 mg cholesterol, 3 g fiber, 5 g protein, 98 mg sodium

Dessert

Raspberry-Topped Brownie Cake

Here's a special treat you can enjoy without guilt. The raspberries are packed with artery-protecting antioxidants and fiber.

8 Servings

- 2 **tablespoons vegetable oil**
- 2 **tablespoons unsweetened cocoa powder**
- 1 **egg**
- ¼ **cup water**
- ¾ **cup sugar**
- ½ **cup flour**
- ¼ **teaspoon baking soda**
- ¼ **teaspoon salt**
- ¼ **cup coarsely chopped pecans**
- 3 **cups raspberries**
- 1 **tablespoon cornstarch mixed with 2 tablespoons water**

1. Preheat the oven to 350°F. Spray an 8-inch round cake pan with nonstick cooking spray. In a large bowl, combine the oil, cocoa powder, egg, ¼ cup of water, ½ cup of the sugar, the flour, baking soda, and salt. Mix until well combined. Fold in the pecans.

2. Pour the batter into the prepared pan and bake for 20 minutes or until a toothpick inserted in the center comes out clean. Cool in the pan on a rack.

3. Meanwhile, in a medium saucepan, combine 1½ cups of the raspberries and the remaining ¼ cup sugar and cook, stirring, for 4 minutes or until the berries are juicy. Stir in the cornstarch mixture and cook, stirring, for 4 minutes or until thickened. Strain through a sieve to remove the seeds. Cool for 10 minutes, then spoon over the brownie base. Arrange the remaining 1½ cups berries on top.

NUTRITION INFORMATION
Per serving: 193 calories, 7 g total fat, 1 g saturated fat, 27 mg cholesterol, 3 g fiber, 3 g protein, 115 mg sodium

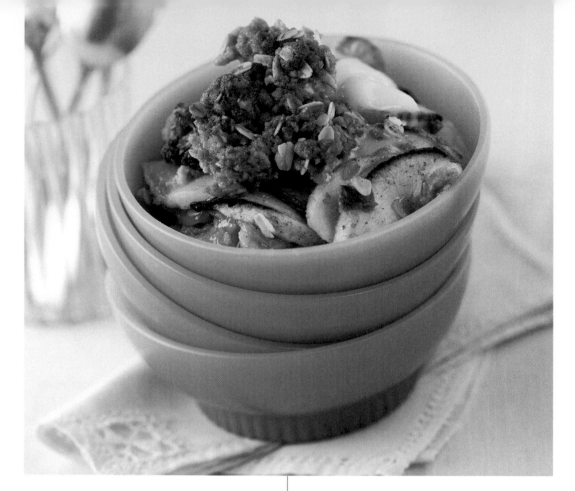

All-Time-Favorite Apple Crisp

Both apples and oatmeal are rich in soluble fiber, which helps lower cholesterol. Indulge in this dessert, and you'll add a serving of fruit to your total for the day.

12 Servings

- 2 **tablespoons plus ½ cup packed light brown sugar**
- 2 **tablespoons plus ⅓ cup all-purpose flour**
- 1 **teaspoon cinnamon**
- I **teaspoon salt**
- 1 **vanilla bean (about 5 inches long) or 1 teaspoon vanilla extract**
- 3 **tablespoons fresh lemon juice**
- 3 **pounds baking apples**
- ½ **cup old-fashioned oats**
- 6 **tablespoons cold margarine, cut into pieces**
- 1 **quart frozen nonfat vanilla yogurt**

1. Preheat oven to 350°F. Lightly coat 13- x 9-inch baking dish with nonstick cooking spray. Mix 2 tablespoons brown sugar, 2 tablespoons flour, ½ teaspoon cinnamon, and ¼ teaspoon salt in food processor bowl. Cut vanilla bean in half lengthwise with paring knife. Scrape out seeds with the back of knife. Add to food processor and pulse to combine, about 10 seconds. Or put in medium bowl and work with hands until well mixed.

2. Put lemon juice in large bowl. Peel apples and cut into ¼-inch slices (you need about 7 cups). Add to bowl, tossing with juice frequently. Sprinkle with brown sugar mixture and toss until evenly coated. Spread in baking dish.

3. Combine oats, remaining brown sugar, remaining flour, remaining cinnamon, and remaining salt in medium bowl. Using your fingers, work margarine into flour mixture until coarse crumbs appear. Sprinkle over apples. Bake until topping is golden and apples are tender, about 40 minutes. Serve with scoops of frozen yogurt.

NUTRITION INFORMATION
Per serving: 266 calories, 6.5 g total fat, 1 g saturated fat, 1 mg cholesterol, 3 g fiber, 5 g protein, 308 mg sodium

Chocolate Chip-Oatmeal Cookies

With half the fat of traditional chocolate chip cookies and an added fiber boost from oatmeal, these goodies will still vanish fast.

Makes 36

- 1 **cup all-purpose flour**
- ½ **teaspoon baking soda**
- ½ **teaspoon salt**
- 1 **cup old-fashioned oats**
- 4 **tablespoons margarine**
- ⅔ **cup packed light brown sugar**
- ½ **cup granulated sugar**
- 1 **large egg**
- 1½ **teaspoons vanilla**
- ⅓ **cup reduced-fat sour cream**
- ¾ **cup semisweet chocolate chips**

1. Preheat oven to 375°F. Line two large baking sheets with parchment paper. Whisk flour, baking soda, and salt in medium bowl. Stir in oats.

2. Cream margarine, brown sugar, and granulated sugar in large bowl with electric mixer at high speed until well blended. Add egg and vanilla and beat until light yellow and creamy, about 3 minutes. Blend in sour cream with wooden spoon, then flour mixture all at once, just until combined (don't overmix or the cookies may become tough). Stir in chocolate chips.

3. Drop dough by heaping teaspoonfuls 2 inches apart onto baking sheets. Bake cookies until golden, about 10 minutes. Cool on baking sheets 2 minutes, then transfer to wire racks and cool completely. Store in airtight container for up to 2 weeks or freeze for up to 3 months.

NUTRITION INFORMATION
Per cookie: 85 calories, 2.5 g total fat, 1 g saturated fat, 7 mg cholesterol, 0.5 g fiber, 1 g protein, 70 mg sodium

Walnut Shortbread

Shortbread is usually made with butter, but this one features a mixture of ground walnuts, olive oil, and walnut oil instead.

8 Servings (16 wedges)

- ⅔ **cup walnuts**
- ¾ **cup all-purpose flour**
- ½ **cup whole-wheat flour**
- ½ **cup confectioners' sugar**
- ¼ **teaspoon salt**
- ¼ **cup walnut oil**
- ¼ **cup light olive oil**
- 1½ **teaspoons grated lemon zest**
- 1 **teaspoon vanilla extract**

1. Preheat the oven to 325°F. Toast the walnuts for 7 minutes or until crisp and fragrant. Leave the oven on. Cool the walnuts, then transfer to a food processor with the all-purpose flour and process until the nuts are finely ground.

2. Transfer the flour-walnut mixture to a large bowl. Stir in the whole-wheat flour, confectioners' sugar, and salt. Add the walnut oil, olive oil, lemon zest, and vanilla and stir until well combined.

3. Press the dough onto the bottom of a 9-inch tart pan with a removable bottom. With the tines of a fork, prick the dough. With a sharp knife, score the dough into 16 wedges, cutting almost, but not quite through, to the bottom.

4. Bake for 30 minutes or until crisp and light golden. Check the shortbread after 20 minutes; if it is overbrowning, decrease the oven temperature to 300°F. Remove from the oven and, while the shortbread is still warm, cut the wedges through to the bottom. Cool in the pan on a wire rack.

NUTRITION INFORMATION
Per serving: 273 calories, 19 g total fat, 2 g saturated fat, 0 mg cholesterol, 1.7g fiber, 3 g protein, 73 mg sodium

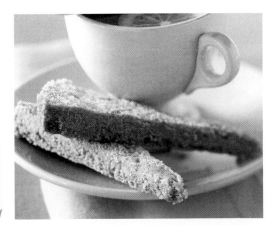

Index

Credits